Literature and Medicine in the Nineteenth-Century Periodical Press

Edinburgh Critical Studies in Romanticism
Series Editors: Ian Duncan and Penny Fielding

Visit our website at: edinburghuniversitypress.com/series-edinburgh-critical-studies-in-romanticism.html

Literature and Medicine in the Nineteenth-Century Periodical Press

Blackwood's Edinburgh Magazine, 1817–1858

Megan Coyer

EDINBURGH
University Press

Edinburgh University Press is one of the leading university presses in the UK. We publish academic books and journals in our selected subject areas across the humanities and social sciences, combining cutting-edge scholarship with high editorial and production values to produce academic works of lasting importance. For more information visit our website: edinburghuniversitypress.com

Edinburgh University Press Ltd
The Tun – Holyrood Road, 12(2f) Jackson's Entry, Edinburgh EH8 8PJ

Typeset in 11/14 Adobe Sabon by
IDSUK (DataConnection) Ltd

A CIP record for this book is available from the British Library

ISBN 978 1 4744 0560 7 (hardback)
ISBN 978 1 4744 0561 4 (webready PDF)
ISBN 978 1 4744 0562 1 (epub)

Contents

Acknowledgements

This work was supported by the Wellcome Trust [097597/Z/11/Z]. I would like to thank the Bodleian Libraries, University of Oxford; the British Library Board; the Harvard Medical Library in the Francis A. Countway Library of Medicine; University of Glasgow Library, Special Collections; the National Library of Scotland; and the Royal Medical Society of Edinburgh for permission to cite and quote from manuscripts in their care. A particular thanks to the librarians in the rare books room at the National Library of Scotland, whose patient assistance enabled me to complete the core research for this book.

I am also grateful to Brill/Rodopi, Pickering & Chatto, and the Association for Scottish Literary Studies for allowing me to reproduce previously published material. An earlier version of a section of Chapter 2 appeared as 'Phrenological Controversy and the Medical Imagination: "A Modern Pythagorean" in *Blackwood's Edinburgh Magazine*' in Megan J. Coyer and David E. Shuttleton (eds), *Scottish Medicine and Literary Culture, 1726–1832* (Amsterdam; New York: Rodopi, 2014), pp. 172–95, and a few sentences from Megan J. Coyer and David E. Shuttleton, 'Introduction: Scottish Medicine and Literary Culture, 1726–1832' (pp. 1–22) appear in the Introduction and in Chapters 2 and 3. An earlier version of Chapter 1 appeared as 'Medical Discourse and Ideology in the *Edinburgh Review*: A Chaldean Exemplar', in Alex Benchimol, Rhona Brown, and David Shuttleton (eds), *Before Blackwood's: Scottish Journalism in the Age of Enlightenment* (London: Pickering & Chatto, 2015), pp. 103–16. A few sentences from my article on 'The Medical Kailyard', *The Bottle Imp* 15 (2014) appear in Chapter 4 and in the Coda.

Like most, this book has been a long time in the making, and I owe a debt of thanks to many who made it possible. A very warm thank you to Professor Kirsteen McCue, who encouraged me to develop this project when it was only one of several ideas scribbled in a note-book towards the end of my doctoral studies. Dr David Shuttleton's mentorship was subsequently invaluable, both in applying for and completing the Wellcome Trust Fellowship that funded the project and in ultimately producing this book. I benefited from many schol-arly conversations with him, and he generously provided comments on several drafts. Likewise, Dr Gavin Miller supported this project at key junctures, most particularly at the fellowship application stage. As co-directors of the Medical Humanities Research Centre at the University of Glasgow, David and Gavin provided a welcoming and intellectually supportive environment for me to develop my ideas. Within the School of Critical Studies at the University of Glasgow, I am grateful to all my colleagues, who make Glasgow a vibrant place to work, but I owe particular thanks to Professor Nigel Leask, Professor Jeremy Smith, Professor Murray Pittock, Dr Rhona Brown, Dr Alex Benchimol, Dr Christine Ferguson, Dr Justin Livingstone, and Professor Gerard Carruthers, each of whom provided support and inspiration at key stages. Thanks also to Dr Pauline Mackay, whose friendship both within and beyond the university has been a sustaining force. I have also benefited from conversations with a range of persons at conferences and meetings, but I owe particu-lar thanks to Professor Lynda Pratt, who graciously assisted me in navigating the correspondence of Robert Southey, and to Professor William Christie, who commented on an early draft of the chapter dedicated to the *Edinburgh Review*.

This book would not have been possible without the belief, enthusiasm and guidance of the series editors, Professor Ian Dun-can and Professor Penny Fielding, who have supported the book from its earliest stages and have continually gone far beyond the call of duty in helping me to see it to fruition. I am also grateful to Adela Rauchova, Jackie Jones, Michelle Houston, and their team at Edinburgh University Press for patiently guiding me through the publishing process, and to the two anonymous readers of the book proposal, who provided invaluable feedback.

I am also eternally grateful to the Wellcome Trust, not only for funding the research fellowship that enabled me to complete the research and writing of this book, but also for supporting and encouraging me at key stages, and I would particularly like to thank David Clayton, Lauren Couch, Leonie Figov, Sophie Hutchison, and

Cecy Marden in this regard. The feedback of the interview panel and the anonymous readers of the fellowship application helped to shape the project, while also giving me the freedom to see where the research might take me.

Lastly, and most importantly, I am grateful for the constant love and support of my family, and in particular, my parents, Ronald and Rebecca, my sister, Rachel, and my brother, Tom. In the course of finishing this book, I joined another family, and I would also like to thank my mother- and father-in-law, Jim and Janette Horn, for their love and support. To my husband, Graham, thank you for all your patience, love and humour. This book is dedicated to you.

Abbreviations

BEM	*Blackwood's Edinburgh Magazine*
EMM	*Edinburgh Monthly Magazine*
EMSJ	*Edinburgh Medical and Surgical Journal*
ER	*Edinburgh Review*
FM	*Fraser's Magazine for Town and Country*
LM	*London Magazine*
LMG	*London Medical Gazette*
MM	*Monthly Magazine*
NLS	National Library of Scotland
NMM	*New Monthly Magazine*
ODNB	*Oxford Dictionary of National Biography*
PJ	*Phrenological Journal and Miscellany*
QR	*Quarterly Review*
SM	*Scots Magazine and Edinburgh Literary Miscellany*

To Graham

Introduction:
Medicine and Blackwoodian
Romanticism

Ours is not, strictly speaking, a medical Journal, though it contains many recipes for a long life and a merry one . . . Yet, though Maga is neither a physician nor a surgeon, nor yet an accoucheur – (though frequently she is Fancy's midwife) – she does not regard with blind eye and deaf ear the medical and surgical world.

Blackwood's Edinburgh Magazine (1830)[1]

In the early nineteenth century, Edinburgh was the leading centre of medical education and research in Britain. It also laid claim to a thriving periodical culture, which served as a significant medium for the dissemination and exchange of medical and literary ideas throughout Britain, the colonies, and beyond. *Literature and Medicine in the Nineteenth-Century Periodical Press* explores the relationship between the medical culture of Romantic-era Scotland and the periodical press by examining several medically-trained contributors to *Blackwood's Edinburgh Magazine*, the most influential and innovative literary periodical of the era. Situating these men's work in relation to developments in medical and periodical culture, the book illustrates how the nineteenth-century periodical press cross-fertilised medical and literary ideas. As we will see, the Romantic periodical press cultivated innovative ideologies, discourses, and literary forms that both reflected and shaped medical culture in the nineteenth century; in the case of *Blackwood's*, the magazine's distinctive Romantic ideology and experimental form enabled the development of an overtly 'literary' and humanistic popular medical culture, which participated in a wider critique of liberal Whig ideology in post-Enlightenment Scotland.

We may begin with a brief example from *Blackwood's* by a non-medical contributor. The quotation at the head of this introduction comes from 'Clark on Climate', a hybrid medico-literary review of the second edition of Dr James Clark's *The Influence of Climate* (1830), attributed to John Wilson (1785–1854), Professor of Moral Philosophy at the University of Edinburgh from 1820 until 1851 and a leading figure in the *Blackwood's* circle. Wilson (in the voice of Christopher North, the fictional editor of *Blackwood's*) relates Clark's findings and recommendations regarding the influence of climate on certain diseases, but also sustains *Blackwood's* general polemic against Whig liberalism. The review begins with a characteristic slight on Francis Jeffrey (1773–1850), the first editor of the *Edinburgh Review*; more specifically, it targets Jeffrey's review of 'Professor M'Culloch's Elements of Political Economy', published in the *Edinburgh Review* in November 1825.[2] From its inception in 1817, *Blackwood's* developed its high Tory Romantic ideology programmatically in opposition to the 'neo-Enlightenment liberalism' of the *Edinburgh Review*.[3] The *Edinburgh's* promotion of Whig political economy as providing 'a scientific basis for Reform' was a particular target,[4] and in a pervasive counter-Enlightenment polemic, *Blackwood's* portrayed the science of political economy as bereft of humane feeling and also inimical to the creative arts. Jeffrey, however, in his review of M'Culloch, reconceptualises political economy as enabling the 'higher and more precious enjoyments' of the 'spiritual' part of our nature.[5] He begins with a binary declaration mocked by Wilson in 'Clark on Climate' – 'MAN, after all, has but a Soul and a Body; – and we can only make him happy by ministering to the wants of the one or the other' – and argues that political economy does, at least indirectly, minister to both.[6] By making the satisfaction of more basic bodily needs and comforts more efficient, according to Jeffrey's formulation, the science creates leisure time and thus encourages the production of the fine arts, which in turn promotes the 'moral and intellectual improvement' of wider society.[7]

Wilson turns Jeffrey's argument on its head, collapsing his hierarchical distinction between the needs of the 'Soul' and the 'Body'. If Jeffrey saw the fine arts as the product of satisfied and thus leisured bodies, Wilson presents artistic production and consumption as essential to bodily health. While promising to summarise Clark's treatise, such that '[i]nvalids – valetudinarians – may thus purchase the advice of an eminent physician for half-a-crown', Wilson notes that they receive

> along with it, a few other prescriptions for various complaints, by one who confines himself chiefly to private practice, and visits poor people unfee'd – Christopher North, who has been a D.D. for upwards of half a century, has attended consultations with Drs Heberden and Hunter – and was brought up at the knees of those Galen [sic] and Hippocrates, the MUNROES.[8]

This extract plays on the medicalised character of North, who was famous for suffering from rheumatism and a gouty toe (and for complaining about it in his reviews), and also sustains a running joke on the healing powers of *Blackwood's* itself.

In a spoof article of 1823, supposedly taken from the *Edinburgh Medical and Surgical Journal*, *Blackwood's* is presented as a cure for Whiggish tendencies, as 'one of the best stimulants to nervous energy with which we are acquainted'. The authors recommend that 'those to whom the public health is of importance . . . give it a fair trial, particularly in *Delirium Constitutionale, D. Taxator, D. Nobilitas, D. Agraria, D. Infidelitas,* and other species of this tantalizing disease'.[9] In this case, the 'mental' stimulation of *Blackwood's* is more effective than the *materia medica*. This macrocosmic appeal to the stimulating powers of *Blackwood's* is paralleled by North's own therapeutic relationship with the magazine. Taking on the North pseudonym, which was by no means the exclusive property of Wilson, William Maginn writes:

> You are acquainted with the nature of my malady, and may well wonder how I can possibly survive it in this metropolis of pharmacy. It is indeed a difficult thing for a sick man to keep alive in a city, where, besides a regular vomitory for doctors of medicine, there are at least 417 graduates of physic, resident and stationary, not to mention the subordinate rank and file of the faculty.[10]

North declares he avoids the doctors at all costs, and '[i]nstead of looking over their pothooks and hangers' he spends his 'time in writing articles which delight the world, or in reading books which delight myself'.[11] If not the magazine, then a ride on top of a mail coach, enables him to declare:

Why, our crutch is now altogether unnecessary. Our toe is painless as if made of timber, yet as steel elastic. Gout, who certainly mounted the mail with us in Prince's Street, has fallen off the roof. . . . No more of that revolutionary, constitution-shaking, radical, French eau-medicinal. A few gulps of Tweedsmuir air have made us quite a young elderly gentleman.[12]

Physic is here equated with 'unnatural' revolutionary politics, while a Wordsworthian return to nature restores health.[13] In a prototypically Romantic gesture against conformity, *Blackwood's* also dismisses regular habits as ineffective for maintaining health. Wilson's review of *Sure Methods of Improving Health, and Prolonging Life, &c. By a Physician* (1827), entitled 'Health and Longevity', includes a table comparing the miserly recommendations of the physician (who is deemed the 'Old Woman') with the decadent fare consumed by Blackwoodian authors (familiar to any reader of the *Noctes Ambrosianæ*). Instead of the Old Woman's prescription of reading aloud to promote pulmonary circulation, North suggests that you 'burst out into a guffaw that startles the Castle rock – and then, letting down the lattice, return to your article, which, like the haggis of the Director-General, is indeed a Roarer'.[14]

The development of the North character and his celebration of the robust embodiment maintained by any Blackwoodian contributor, who 'with a sound Tory Church and King stomach and constitution cannot overeat himself', was part of a unifying voice of 'belligerent High Toryism' that brought cohesion to a magazine often distinguished by its constant variety.[15] Jon Klancher's seminal study views the major periodicals and literary magazines of the Romantic period as shaping new reading audiences through such 'powerful transauthorial' discourses, and cites both *Blackwood's* and the *Edinburgh Review* as working to shape a new middle-class reading public through their role as 'a collective interpreter mapping out the cultural physiognomy of Britain'.[16] However, while the writers of the *Edinburgh* consistently turned to political economy, *Blackwood's*, in stark contrast, emphasised the importance of 'natural', and importantly, embodied feelings in interpreting society, politics, and culture.

The 'Preface' to the January 1826 number reflects upon the Blackwoodian revolution in literature and in politics:

A warm, enthusiastic, imaginative, and, at the same time, philosophical spirit, breathed through every article. Authors felt that they were understood and appreciated, and readers were delighted to have their own uncorrupted feelings authorized and sanctioned. . . . People were encouraged to indulge their emotions, that they might be brought to know their nature. That long icy chill was shook off their fancies and imaginations, and here, too, in Criticism as in Politics, they began to feel, think, and speak, like free men.[17]

The magazine's continual recurrence to its healing powers, based on its embodied effect on readers and contributors, works to authenticate this declared revolution. In contrast, it repeatedly portrays political economy and sceptical philosophy as the products of abstract intellectual reasoning and hence devoid of feeling. John Gibson Lockhart (1794–1854), another key player in the early years of *Blackwood's*, in a satirical article on political economy in November 1822, echoes the cold reasoning of Swift's 'modest proposal' by reporting that a 'Professor Bumgroschen' has suggested that, since the essence of political economy is to make persons useful to the wider community, persons should be as useful in death as in life: they should first be dissected for the benefit of medical science, then displayed in a museum for the benefit of public education, and finally sent to the 'College of Arts and Manufactures' to be transformed into useful material objects.[18] Lockhart's article also indicates how medical science might be aligned with political economy in terms of their shared investment in the infamous 'march of intellect' promoted by Whig ideology. However, *Blackwood's* was not 'anti-medical'. Rather, as this book will detail, the magazine endorsed a medical culture that valued embodied human feeling and imagination (while also paradoxically drawing attention to the potentially problematic nature of an aestheticised medical gaze). Through its distinctive Romantic ideology and its 'innovative mixture of literary forms and discourses'[19] *Blackwood's* enabled the development of new forms and modes of popular medical writing as well as the construction of an idealised figure of the literary medical man for the wider reading public of the nineteenth century.

Lockhart's Blackwoodian spin-off project, *Peter's Letters to his Kinsfolk* (1819), offers a book-length account of the magazine's oppositional Romantic ideology. Following the tradition of Tobias

Smollett's character Matthew Bramble, the epistolary author of the text, the Welsh physician Dr Peter Morris, M.D., provides a cultural biography of Scotland in a series of letters to familiar correspondents. The Dr Morris character, like Christopher North, is fictitiously developed as a flesh-and-blood human individual. A review of the nonexistent first edition of *Peter's Letters* in *Blackwood's* – a hoax designed to promote the sales of the 'second edition' – praises Morris for his capability 'of feeling so many different sorts of things, and of doing so much justice to what he does feel'.[20] In his critical study of Lockhart, Francis Hart identifies Morris's stance as a 'Romantic cultural observer' – an active, embodied interpreter of what he encounters on his journey through Scotland – and points to Morris's reaction to one of the Reverend Thomas Chalmers' sermons as the 'thematic centre of the entire book'.[21] Morris declares:

> I have never heard, either in England, or Scotland, or in any other country, any preacher whose eloquence is capable of producing an effect so strong and irresistible as his. . . . I was proud to feel my hardened nerves creep and vibrate, and my blood freeze and boil while he spake – as they were wont to do in the early innocent years, when unquestioning enthusiasm had as yet caught no lessons of chillness from the jealousies of discernment, the delights of comparison, and the example of the unimaginative world.[22]

In contrast, Morris accuses the *Edinburgh Review* and its devoted cohort of young Whigs, 'the legitimate progeny of the sceptical philosophers of the last age', of propagating cold, self-serving critical reasoning and 'a system of scepticism . . . entirely irreconcilable with the notion of any fervent love and attachment for a religion, which is, above all other things, the religion of feeling'.[23] Rather than active, embodied interpreters, these young Whigs passively reiterate the superficial knowledge gained through reading the *Edinburgh Review*, continuously replicating a false, infidel national culture divorced from 'the true ornaments of our nature'.[24] According to Lockhart, intellectual reasoning is universal and modes of feeling peculiar to nations and cultures; Ian Duncan aptly deems this formulation to be an early version of 'the notorious "Caledonian Antisyzygy" or dissociation of sensibility, in its classic definition of a split between intellect and feeling'.[25] Importantly, in order for Lockhart to declare a transformative reconstitution of an organic national culture through the glorification of history and the 'hero as man of letters' (in Lockhart's case, Scott) who 'restores, in his own example, the organic, synecdochic relation between individual and society that constitutes national character', he has to first provide evidence that such a culture has truly been disrupted.[26] As we will see, Scottish medicine, political economy, and sceptical philosophy all provided apt targets, but like national culture, medical culture was also primed for transformative reconstitution, in which the 'severed faculties of reason and sentiment' might be reunited through an engagement with literary culture.[27]

The development of *Blackwood's* distinctive Romantic ideology occurred when Scottish medicine had reached a pivotal point in its development. Since the establishment of the medical faculty at the University of Edinburgh in 1726, medicine had been at the heart of an ethos of improvement and progress – the 'march of intellect' associated with the Scottish Enlightenment. While leading historians and critics such as Hugh Trevor-Roper and Nicolas Phillipson have identified moral philosophy, history, and political economy as the core subjects of the Enlightenment curriculum and the 'social behaviour of mankind' as its central concern, and the Union of 1707 as the Scottish Enlightenment's primary historical catalyst, Roger Emerson has instead looked to Newtonian science and Baconian inductive philosophy as internal driving forces.[28] For Paul Wood, also, '[s]cience and medicine were central to, and in some cases the driving force behind, the intellectual changes encompassed by the term "the Scottish Enlightenment"'.[29] As L. S. Jacyna notes, 1789 – the year in which the influential medical teacher and theorist William Cullen (1710–90) retired from his prestigious position as chair of the practice of medicine – is traditionally cited as the end of a 'Golden Age' of medicine in Edinburgh.[30] However, Jacyna goes on to reveal the first half of the nineteenth century to be a period of substantial innovation. Key figures such as Andrew Duncan, junior (1773–1832) and John Thomson (1765–1846) worked against the Tory-dominated Town Council (which controlled university appointments at Edinburgh until the Universities (Scotland) Act of 1858) and a medical faculty populated by nepotistic dynasties to establish new chairs that reflected the rapidly changing needs of society and the medical profession in the nineteenth century.[31]

As I will fully detail in Chapter 1, the *Edinburgh Review*, in its early years, was a major voice in the move towards medical reform in Scotland. In his 1825 review of M'Culloch Jeffrey reflects upon the success of this reform – the fruitfulness of 'the *division of labour*' in the medical faculty – to voice retrospective support for M'Culloch's attempt to found a separate chair of political economy at Edinburgh.[32] Wilson had opposed the scheme, not only because it threatened to place his 'inveterate enemy, the local Whig of Whigs . . . pleasantly known to Blackwood's gang as "the Stot"' (i.e. M'Culloch) in a position of political power, but also because the proposed chair would have encroached upon his own subject matter, since political economy was traditionally part of the curriculum of moral philosophy at Edinburgh.[33] Wilson's criticism of Jeffrey's review of M'Culloch in the context of reviewing a medical text is thus telling, representing as it does a wider reappropriation of medical culture for the conservative cause.

Most studies to date have focused on the association of Scottish medicine and medical science with improvement and reform.[34] The practical, relatively affordable, and non-denominational medical education available at the University of Edinburgh is considered to be a main driving force behind the professionalisation of medicine in Britain as well as a major component in the production of the Victorian cultural hegemony of liberal bourgeois capitalism, wherein merit overtook the primacy of rank.[35] Adrian Desmond's *The Politics of Evolution: Morphology, Medicine, and Reform in Radical London* (1989) views the Edinburgh medical scene in the 1820s as a feeder pool for London radicalism in the 1830s, and as paving the way for Charles Darwin's articulation of 'a Malthusian science for the rising industrial-professional middle classes'.[36] In *Philosophic Whigs: Medicine, Science, and Citizenship in Edinburgh, 1789–1848* (1994) Jacyna provides the most detailed study of Scottish medical culture in the first half of the nineteenth century. Jacyna represents the 'philosophic Whigs', namely, the surgeon and lecturer on physiology John Allen (1771–1843), John Thomson, and his son, Allen Thomson (1809–84), as motivated by the virtues of civic humanism in their wide-ranging medical, literary and scientific pursuits, which also reflected their progressive political visions for society. Jacyna sees Dugald Stewart (1753–1828), 'the most influential interpreter of Enlightenment thought for the new generation', as foundational for the 'philosophic Whigs', in particular because of his advocacy of a liberal education, underpinned by the study of moral philosophy, to counteract the limitations of specialism and division of labour.[37] However, in considering the specific context of the *Edinburgh Review*, this understanding of Whig ideology should be slightly amended. Jeffrey departed from Stewart's teachings in two key articles of 1804 and 1810 and, according to George Davie, joined with William Cobbett and the Utilitarians in declaring that 'in the new conditions of the nineteenth century, mental philosophy was not so useful socially and educationally as the earlier Scottish Enlightenment had thought'.[38] Rather, for Jeffrey, 'experimental sciences like chemistry were making an indispensable and indisputable contribution to the economic advance'.[39] Anand Chitnis views this shift as part of the *Edinburgh*'s revision of Enlightenment thought – its 'modifications of Scottish philosophical education in what was regarded as a more utilitarian age'.[40] Meanwhile Michelle Faubert has fruitfully carried Jacyna's definition of the 'philosophic Whigs' forward in her study of nineteenth-century 'psychologist-poets', most of whom studied at Edinburgh. She emphasises the 'Whiggish' character of the Scottish medical schools and the tendency of 'Scottish Whigs' to encourage 'a diversity of interests and areas of expertise as insurance against intellectual tyranny and conservativism'.[41] The figure of the physician as man-of-letters, who promotes his professional identity and disseminates information to 'all classes and types of people' through his writings, becomes a direct product of Whig politics and the Scottish Enlightenment, as well as a Foucauldian asserter of disciplinary power.[42]

The other side of the story – that belonging to Scottish Romanticism and the high Tory politics of *Blackwood's* – has yet to be told, and it is a story that involves the development of a humanistic and overtly 'literary' popular medical culture in the periodical press that was part of a wider reaction to Whig liberalism. In essence, I contend that, if the early nineteenth-century interpreters and popularisers of the values of the Scottish Enlightenment – the *Edinburgh* reviewers – contributed to what would become the liberal hegemony of Victorian society, with its emphasis on professionalism, utilitarianism and increasingly reductive scientific principles, the network of writers surrounding *Blackwood's* developed the foundations for the critique of that hegemony. To examine this thesis, this book recovers a circle of medical writers all of whom contributed to *Blackwood's* during its most influential years, between its founding in 1817 and the death of William Blackwood in 1834.[43] This grouping includes: William Pulteney Alison (1790–1859), D. M. Moir (1798–1851), Robert Macnish (1802–37), Samuel Warren (1807–77), William Dunlop (1792–1848), John Howison (1797–1859), Robert Ferguson (1799–1865) and Robert Gooch (1784–1830).[44] Importantly, these writers had wide-ranging medical and literary careers and also contributed to other periodicals, such as the *Quarterly Review*, the *Scots Magazine*, and *Fraser's Magazine for Town and Country*, as well as specialist medical journals such as the *London Medical Gazette*. However, *Blackwood's* serves as a common context for their participation in the development of modes of popular medical writing and engagement with key ideas that became part of an emergent nineteenth-century medical humanism. Like the Romantic cultural nationalism of *Blackwood's*, this medical humanism was reactionary in its politics and depended upon 'division as its empirical foundation' – a perceived disconnect between intellectual development and spiritual core.[45] Building upon Philip Connell's claim that 'nineteenth-century political economy, and the debate on its legitimacy, scope, and function, played a formative role in the emergence of the idea of "culture" itself, as a humanistic or spiritual resource resistant to the intellectual enervation produced by modern, commercial societies', I argue that these writers produced a body of popular medical writing that worked to counter what Connell terms the perceived 'opposition between literature, aesthetics, and feeling, on the one hand; and science, utility, and reason, on the other', which was concurrently developing in the nineteenth century.[46]

A significant aspect of this was the formulation of the physician or surgeon as man-of-letters and humanitarian, who could rise above the commercial forces of industrial society to endorse a theory and practice of medicine based upon intuitive moral and religious feelings. North's long-running critique of medical professionals (and their 'revolutionary' physic), for example, is balanced against his portrayal of the traditional, 'gentlemanly' physician-figure. In 'Health and Longevity', he provides full descriptions of the 'Three Kinds' of physicians: 'your man of education – your scholar and your gentleman – who is as open, honest, and sincere at your bedside, as at your dinner-table'; 'your Old Woman' who is over-anxious and thus

overly medicates and acts as a 'radical reformer'; and 'your Quack' –
'[h]ard-hearted, coarse, vulgar, greedy, profligate, and unprincipled,
in his unfearing ignorance'.[47] Dr Clark of 'Clark on Climate' is portrayed as the first kind and 'the *beau ideal* of an anti-quack', 'who
knows too well the beatings of the human heart'.[48] Further, while
other doctors wrap all their knowledge 'up in guinea-pills, which it
is often as difficult to purchase as to swallow', Clark has penned a
medical text 'intelligible to the generality of readers, without at all
diminishing the utility of the work to the members of his own profession', and North expresses his 'hope that other physicians will lay
aside the stilts and the veil'.[49] Aptly, this number of *Blackwood's* also
contains the first chapter of Warren's *Passages from the Diary of a
Late Physician*, serialised in the magazine between 1830 and 1837,
which promised to provide the 'secret history' of the medical profession whilst also portraying an ideal moral and religious gentleman
physician-figure – a medical 'man of feeling' and man-of-letters –
who complemented the Tory initiative to develop a popular literature
reflecting conservative values as 'a defence against the impending
social anarchy threatened by the commercial spirit'.[50]

While the Romantic ideology of *Blackwood's* – particularly as
presented in *Peter's Letters to his Kinsfolk* – was defined, in part, in
opposition to the philosophy of Dugald Stewart and his successor,
Thomas Brown (1778–1820), the magazine's emphasis on natural
moral and religious feelings reflects the foundational principles of
the Common Sense school of Scottish philosophy. Morris dismisses
their 'mechanical mode of observation' as 'perhaps better adapted
for throwing light upon the intellectual faculties, and upon the association of ideas, than upon human nature in general', insisting that

> [t]he scope and tendency of the different affections can never be gathered
> from the analyses of particular trains of thought, or by such a micro-
> scopic and divided mode of observation, as that which consists in watch-
> ing the succession of ideas as they arise in the mind.[51]

Instead, we must turn to '[p]oetry and eloquence' and study 'Mr
Wordsworth's small pieces, such as Michael, the Brothers, or the
Idiot Boy' or 'the broken catches of multitudinous feelings, in the
speeches of one such character as Madge Wildfire' to understand
'that most valuable, and perhaps most divine part of our nature'.[52]

Morris's proposed methodology echoes the semiotic theory of perception developed by Thomas Reid (1710–96), the founder of the Common Sense school. Reid distinguished between natural signs, such as gesture and facial expression, the significance of which all persons innately recognised, and artificial signs, such as spoken and written language, the significance of which were culturally transmitted.[53] By 'a kind of natural magic' a person instinctively conceived the significance of these natural signs in the external world, and our eventual understanding of generalised artificial signs was based upon this instinctive knowledge.[54] Reid's second class of natural sign (from which our innate knowledge of the existence of other minds is derived) is said to be the 'foundation of the fine arts', as '[i]n the expressiveness of the arts we hear again the primordial language which we can all understand' while 'the beauty and sublimity of nature is God's mind, so to speak, sensibly present'.[55] Reid's theory was a reactionary attack on the scepticism of David Hume, who unlike Reid, and later Stewart and Brown, did not take mankind's irresistible belief in the external world as a first principle, instilled in man by God.

First principles, instilled by the 'the First Great Cause', were foundational to the Common Sense school, as an inherently Christian philosophy. Some critics have recently turned to the significance of Common Sense philosophy – its simultaneous formulation of an actively processing intuitive mind and endorsement of inductive Baconian practices – in questioning the traditional understanding of Romanticism, promoted by M. H. Abrams, as rooted in German philosophy and inherently anti-empiricist.[56] This move away from the context of Kantian philosophy is crucial for a study of the relationship between *Blackwood's* particular brand of Romanticism and medical culture. For example, in 1858 William Pulteney Alison was still 'anxious to show that the Scottish schools of medicine maintained their connexion with the studies and doctrines of Reid and of Stewart, of Brown, Abercrombie, and Chalmers',[57] and Common Sense philosophy's appeal to 'the First Great Cause' and 'ultimate facts' could enable the reconciliation of medical science and religion that was central to the Blackwoodian engagement with scientific discourses.[58] Further, key medical figures, such as the Edinburgh physician and popular philosopher John Abercrombie (1780–1844), built upon the earlier work of John Gregory (1724–73) to provide an account of intuitive, 'feeling'-based moral and religious impulses, articulated as common to all men in a healthful state, which provided a basis for ethical practice within the school of medicine associated with Common Sense philosophy.

Common Sense philosophy, however, could also problematise the empirical project of nineteenth-century medicine, since, as Gavin Budge indicates, its 'insistence on immaterial intuition as the source of knowledge brings to the fore the problematic nature of the material forms in which intuition is embodied'.[59] In other words, the embodiment of the observing subject is brought into focus. J. H. Alexander has noted that embodiment became a key component of the innovative literary criticism of *Blackwood's*, in which (in contrast to the objective tone of the *Edinburgh Review*) 'critical judgments emerge from concrete situations – from living men reading works under particular circumstances and varying in their reactions'.[60] The characterisation and style of Christopher North are a case in point. However, the emphasis on subjective embodiment could be problematic for physicians and surgeons participating in a medico-scientific culture in which 'mechanical objectivity' was increasingly valued.

Lorraine Daston and Peter Galison have eloquently analysed the process by which concepts associated with professional medico-scientific thinking, such as 'mechanical objectivity', were defined against Romantic concepts of the 'active' mind.[61] They describe the 'divided scientific self, actively willing its own passivity' and '[i]ts polar opposite, equally stereotyped and normalized . . . the artistic self, as militantly subjective as the scientific self was objective'.[62] Michel Foucault's infamous formulation of the medical gaze characterises a similar valuation of objectivity for the growing professional authority of medicine in particular: manifesting 'its virtues only in a double silence: the relative silence of theories, imaginings, and whatever serves as an obstacle to the sensible immediate', the 'neutral' clinical gaze would combine with pathological anatomy to comprise the 'anatomico-clinical' gaze of nineteenth-century medicine.[63] However, while scientific practices, and more importantly, the rhetorical display of scientific practices,[64] were key in establishing the legitimacy of 'regular' versus 'irregular' medical practitioners (a distinction that was only solidified with the Medical Act of 1858 and its creation of a list of registered practitioners), medicine is unique among the modern professions associated with industrial society in the level of emphasis it places on 'credibility and legitimation' gained through interpersonal relationships.[65] As Magali Sarfatti Larson notes, '[i]n a secularized society, the family doctor of old is one of the most direct inheritors of the role of the religious minister or priest'.[66] Wilson makes this comparison explicit in 'Health and Longevity' when he declares his fondness for the 'healing tribe' – for 'Doctors, either of Religion or Medicine'.[67] Tabitha Sparks's recent chronological tracking of novelistic depictions of medical practitioners argues for the dominance of a professionalism based upon a 'ministerial service-ideal rather than a proto-scientific objective [sic]' in the mid-nineteenth century, as exemplified by such idyllic figures as Martineau's Edward Hope in *Deerbrook* (1839) and Dickens's Allan Woodcourt in *Bleak House* (1852–3).[68] My study looks back earlier in the century, to when this idyllic image was only gradually emerging in popular culture, during a period in which the medico-scientific values of the post-Enlightenment period were at times perceived as in conflict with the Romantic literary valuation of subjectivity, individuality, and 'natural' feelings.

Literature and Medicine in the Nineteenth-Century Periodical Press tracks how a group of Tory medical writers, associated with the seminal literary magazine of the Romantic period, negotiated their medico-literary careers in this fraught context, in which the 'two cultures' model of C. P. Snow was consolidating. Arranged thematically within a loosely chronological structure, the book's chapters focus upon individual authors or groups of authors. The opening chapter provides a comparative context by examining key medical figures associated with *Blackwood's* ideological competitor, the *Edinburgh Review*, and sets the scene by illustrating the relationship between Scottish medicine and the periodical press before the founding of *Blackwood's*. The second chapter focuses on the 'tale of terror' as a key genre in the early years of the magazine. It examines how the sensational Gothic subjectivities associated with this hybrid 'medico-popular' genre both contributed to and problematised the medico-literary projects of contributors such as Howison, Dunlop, and Macnish. The latter two were also associated with the rise of medical jurisprudence and the phrenological movement in Scotland – two fields that valorised an objective standpoint. Chapters 3 and 4 show how Moir and Warren drew upon the ideologies, discourses, and literary forms of the Romantic periodical press to promote an idealistic image of the nineteenth-century medical practitioner, who stood above the dehumanising 'march of intellect' and was driven rather by the medico-philosophical concept of sympathy and the moral and religious 'feelings' valued by the Common Sense school of Scottish philosophy. The emphasis placed on moral and religious feelings in *Blackwood's* also shaped its contribution to the heated popular debates surrounding the rise of public health in the nineteenth century. Chapter 5 examines the construction of the 'political medicine' of Alison and Gooch, based upon the inherent conflict between their medical ideologies and Malthusian political economy, and its development and popular dissemination through *Blackwood's*. In this chapter Ferguson's contributions on public health to the *Quarterly Review* provide a fruitful contrast with Alison and Gooch's *Blackwood's* writings. A coda to the book reflects upon the lasting contribution of *Blackwood's* to nineteenth-century medical humanism by analysing a medical tale by Sir Arthur Conan Doyle, the key Scottish physician-writer of the late nineteenth century, and what I have elsewhere called the 'medical kailyard' of John Watson (1850–1907), published under his pseudonym 'Ian Maclaren'.[69] In contrast to Sparks, who highlights the depiction of medical practitioners in *fin-de-siècle* literature as 'hyper-rational scientists', 'detached from the common feelings of the civilised, feeling person', I emphasise the concurrent reaction against such stereotypes, particularly within the Scottish literary scene.[70]

The end-date for the main body of the text is 1858 (not including the coda). This has been dictated in part by the fact that all the medical writers that form the backbone of this study are either deceased or no longer publishing by this date. Further, the passing of the Medical Act of 1858 marks the point at which Scottish medicine becomes less distinctive from that of the UK as a whole. Finally, it enables the study to remain within the pre-Darwinian era and hence to avoid the problem of trying to do justice, in the limited space available, to very disparate material and formations on either side of a major intellectual watershed.

This is not an exhaustive examination of the medical content of all periodicals to which these writers contributed. Rather, their own contributions are examined within the wider discursive frameworks, ideological contexts, and stylistic conventions of the periodical press, since a key point of interest is how they drew upon these contexts and conventions in forwarding their medico-literary projects. In this I follow Mark Parker's simultaneously abstracted and individuated approach to the study of popular periodicals.[71] Wider developments within Scottish medicine, and particularly academic medicine, provide the cultural context for examining these figures; however, the book is not intended to be a new history of Scottish medicine, but rather a study of a particular literary aspect of a prevailing medical culture and a group of medical writers associated with the Romantic periodical press. It is intended to contribute to our understanding of Scottish Romanticism, the pervasive and ideologically loaded medical content of the nineteenth-century popular periodical press (which has been brought to light by projects such as 'Science in the Nineteenth-Century Periodical' (1999–2007)), and the pivotal importance of the Romantic period in the development of medical humanism.

While critical awareness of the key place of medical culture in informing Romantic literary ideologies and practices has increased in recent years (Sharon Ruston's *Creating Romanticism: Case Studies in the Literature, Science and Medicine of the 1790s* (2013) is exemplary), there has been little recognition of the salience of the Romantic period not only for the formulation of the 'two cultures' model but also for redemptive counter-discourses of medical humanism that bridged not only the 'literary' and the 'medical' but also popular and professional spheres. Critics such as Noel Jackson and James Robert Allard have shown that the figure of the poet-physician, developed by both Wordsworth and Keats, acted as a source of healing, recuperating social consensus via aesthetic culture, and the Romantic poet-physician is read as challenging emergent disciplinary divisions and representing the embodied, imaginative sympathy necessary for the alleviation of suffering.[72] This book, however, turns primarily to the Scottish context (the centre of British medical teaching and research) to argue that the ideological conflicts that brought forth Scottish Romanticism (as heralded by the founding of *Blackwood's*) also brought forth a recuperative humanistic popular medical culture. Importantly, this culture was not produced and contained just in *Blackwood's*. It fundamentally changed the ways in which the literary magazines of the nineteenth century engaged with medicine, and played an important role in formulating a conception of medical humanism that has maintained its currency well into the twenty-first century.

Notes

1. [John Wilson], 'Clark on Climate', *BEM*, 28 (August 1830), 372–81 (p. 372). Attributions in *Blackwood's* have been made based on *The Wellesley Index to Victorian Periodicals* and Alan Lang Strout's *A Bibliography of Articles in Blackwood's Edinburgh Magazine, Volumes I through XVIII: 1817–1825* (Lubbock: Texas Tech Press, 1959).
2. [Wilson], 'Clark on Climate', p. 372.
3. Duncan, *Scott's Shadow*, p. 27.
4. Ibid. p. 26.
5. [Francis Jeffrey], 'Political Economy', *ER*, 43 (November 1825), 1–23 (p. 3, p. 1).
6. Ibid. p. 1.
7. Ibid. p. 2. For a fuller reading of this review article, see Connell, *Romanticism, Economics, and the Question of 'Culture'*, pp. 93–101.
8. [Wilson], 'Clark on Climate', p. 373.
9. [Mr. Starke], 'Vox Populi', *BEM*, 13 (January 1823), 125–38 (p. 128).
10. [William Maginn], 'Letter to Pierce Egan, Esq.', *BEM*, 8 (March 1821), 671–7 (p. 671).
11. Ibid. p. 671.
12. [John Wilson], 'Streams', *BEM*, 19 (April 1826), 375–403 (p. 388).
13. Ibid. p. 388.
14. [John Wilson], 'Health and Longevity', *BEM*, 23 (January 1828), 96–111 (p. 111).
15. [John Wilson], 'The Traveller's Oracle', *BEM*, 22 (October 1827), 445–65 (p. 455); Morrison and Roberts, '"A character so various, and yet so indisputably its own"', in Morrison and Roberts (eds), *Romanticism and Blackwood's Magazine*, p. 1.
16. Klancher, *The Making of English Reading Audiences*, p. 52.
17. [John Wilson, John Galt, David Robinson, and William Maginn], 'Preface', *BEM*, 19 (January 1826), i–xxx (p. xxii).
18. [J. G. Lockhart], 'Political Economy', *BEM*, 12 (November 1822), 525–30 (p. 527).
19. Duncan, *Scott's Shadow*, p. 27.
20. [J. G. Lockhart], 'A Few Farther Strictures on "Peter's Letters to his Kinsfolk", with Extracts from that Popular Work', *BEM*, 4 (March 1819), 745–52 (p. 751).
21. Hart, *Lockhart as Romantic Biographer*, p. 54, p. 68.
22. [Lockhart], *Peter's Letters to his Kinsfolk*, vol. 3, pp. 273–4.
23. Ibid. vol. 2, p. 128, p. 136.
24. Ibid. vol. 2, p. 129.
25. Duncan, '*Blackwood's* and Romantic Nationalism', p. 78.

26. Ibid. p. 72.
27. Ibid. p. 76.
28. Wood and Withers, 'Introduction', in Withers and Wood (eds), *Science and Medicine in the Scottish Enlightenment*, pp. 1–16; Trevor-Roper, 'The Scottish Enlightenment', p. 1639. Key articles by Phillipson include: 'Culture and Society in the Eighteenth-Century Province: The Case of Edinburgh and the Scottish Enlightenment', 'Towards a Definition of the Scottish Enlightenment', and 'The Scottish Enlightenment'.
29. Wood, 'Science in the Scottish Enlightenment', p. 95.
30. Jacyna, *Philosophic Whigs*, p. 1.
31. See also, Rosner, *Medical Education in the Age of Improvement*; Lawrence, 'The Edinburgh Medical School and the End of the "Old Thing" 1790–1830'.
32. [Jeffrey], 'Political Economy', p. 21. Ironically, Jeffrey, M'Culloch's friend and political ally, was largely responsible for the proposal's failure. See O'Brien, *J. R. McCulloch*, p. 33.
33. Swann, *Christopher North <John Wilson>*, p. 174.
34. For example, see Hamilton, *The Healers*, pp. 91–145; Hamilton, 'The Scottish Enlightenment and Clinical Medicine'; Rosner, *Medical Education in the Age of Improvement*; Tröhler, "To Improve the Evidence of Medicine"; Dingwall, *A History of Scottish Medicine*, pp. 108–52.
35. Corfield, *Power and the Professions in Britain*, p. 159; see also Rosner, *Medical Education in the Age of Improvement*. This latter thesis is most clearly articulated by Chitnis in *The Scottish Enlightenment & Early Victorian English Society*.
36. Desmond, *The Politics of Evolution*, p. 410.
37. Duncan, *Scott's Shadow*, p. 26; Jacyna, *Philosophic Whigs*, pp. 36–48.
38. Davie, *The Scottish Enlightenment and Other Essays*, p. 71.
39. Ibid. p. 71.
40. Chitnis, *The Scottish Enlightenment: A Social History*, p. 214. For extracts from Jeffrey's debate with Stewart, see Flynn, *Enlightenment Scotland*, pp. 76–88.
41. Faubert, *Rhyming Reason*, p. 4.
42. Ibid. p. 5.
43. I define 'medical writers' as writers who underwent medical or surgical training, and of this grouping, only Samuel Warren was not also an active practitioner. On his claims to medical training, see Chapter 4, p. 132.

44. Two additional medical contributors who might have been included in this study are Kenneth Macleay (*fl.* 1789–1829) and Charles Badham (1780–1845); however, after an initial perusal of their contributions to *Blackwood's* and wider medico-literary careers, I decided to omit them on the grounds of minimal involvement with the magazine and the Romantic periodical press more broadly.
45. Duncan, *Scott's Shadow*, p. 61.
46. Connell, *Romanticism, Economics, and the Question of 'Culture'*, p. 7, p. 11.
47. [Wilson], 'Health and Longevity', p. 98, p. 106.
48. [Wilson], 'Clark on Climate', p. 373.
49. Ibid. p. 372, p. 381.
50. [Samuel Warren], 'Chap. I. Early Struggles', *BEM*, 28 (August 1830), 322–38 (p. 322); Connell, *Romanticism, Economics, and the Question of 'Culture'*, p. 237.
51. [Lockhart], *Peter's Letters*, vol. 1, p. 175, p. 176.
52. Ibid. pp. 176–7.
53. For a critical overview of Reid's definition of natural versus artificial signs, see Grave, *The Scottish Philosophy of Common Sense*, pp. 151–89.
54. Lehrer, 'Beyond Impressions and Ideas: Hume v. Reid', p. 119.
55. Grave, *The Scottish Philosophy of Common Sense*, p. 154.
56. Budge (ed.), *Romantic Empiricism*; Jackson, *Science and Sensation in Romantic Poetry*; Budge, *Romanticism, Medicine and the Natural Supernatural*.
57. W. P. Alison, 'The Science of Life: its Study and Connections', *British Medical Journal*, 86 (21 August 1858), 699–703 (p. 699).
58. On the reconciliation of science and religion in early *Blackwood's*, see Christie, '*Blackwood's Edinburgh Magazine* in the Scientific Culture of Early Nineteenth-Century Edinburgh', in Morrison and Roberts (eds), *Romanticism and Blackwood's Magazine*, pp. 125–36.
59. Budge, *Romanticism, Medicine and the Natural Supernatural*, p. 16.
60. Alexander, '*Blackwood's*: Magazine as Romantic Form', p. 63.
61. 'Mechanical Objectivity' and 'The Scientific Self', in Daston and Galison, *Objectivity*, pp. 115–90, pp. 191–251.
62. Ibid. p. 246.
63. Foucault, *The Birth of the Clinic*, p. 132, p. 166.
64. Shortt, 'Physicians, Science, and Status'. For a broader examination of the performative aspects of medical professionalism in the nineteenth century, see Brown, *Performing Medicine*.
65. Larson, *The Rise of Professionalism*, p. 22.

66. Ibid. p. 22.
67. [Wilson], 'Health and Longevity', p. 96.
68. Sparks, *The Doctor in the Victorian Novel*, p. 37.
69. See Coyer, 'The Medical Kailyard'.
70. Sparks, *The Doctor in the Victorian Novel*, p. 22, p. 17.
71. Parker, *Literary Magazines and British Romanticism*.
72. Jackson, *Science and Sensation in Romantic Poetry*, pp. 132–62; Allard, *Romanticism, Medicine, and the Poet's Body*, pp. 87–110.

Chapter 1

Medical Discourse and Ideology in the *Edinburgh Review*

'MEDICAL subjects ought in general, we think, to be left to the Medical Journals.'

Edinburgh Review (1806)[1]

In his classic essay on 'Lay Medical Knowledge in the Eighteenth Century: The Evidence of the *Gentleman's Magazine*' (1985), Roy Porter cites this striking declaration as indicative of 'a growing intellectual division of labour amongst both opinion-producers and opinion-consumers, in which medicine was being set aside for specialists'.[2] As such, the review article is seen to represent the nineteenth-century revision of the eighteenth-century public sphere – a move away from the 'notion that men of differing ranks could discourse within it on all subjects on equal terms, through the authenticating token of Enlightenment rationality'.[3] However, within the early nineteenth-century Edinburgh literary marketplace, local commercial factors were also at play: the article was co-authored by Jeffrey and Andrew Duncan, junior, and its appearance shortly after the launching of Duncan's own specialist periodical, the *Edinburgh Medical and Surgical Journal*, in 1805 is most probably not a coincidence.[4] The *Edinburgh Medical and Surgical Journal* was also published by Archibald Constable (an advertisement for the new medical journal may be found in the *Edinburgh Review* of October 1805), and it was not to Constable's or his editors' advantage for two of his most successful periodical publications to compete with one another.

Medical content in the *Edinburgh Review* does markedly decline following the 1806 statement, with coverage only extending to medical topics of significant public concern (such as vaccination, malaria, contagious fever, and the treatment of the mentally ill) and also those of particular interest to chemists, physiologists or anatomists. However, the prevalence of medical content and the importance of medical contributors in the early years of the *Edinburgh* has yet to be fully recognised, and this chapter examines medical discourses and ideologies in the *Edinburgh* to set up a comparative context for examining the relationship of their primary ideological competitor – *Blackwood's Edinburgh Magazine* – to medical culture. I argue that the reforming and professionalising rhetoric of the *Edinburgh* emerged, in part, from medico-scientific culture and was harnessed by medical contributors and carried forward in Constable's medical journal, which, as David Hamilton notes, had a 'similar format' to the *Edinburgh Review* and 'a similar authority in medical circles'.[5] As we will see, the move away from including specialist medical content in the *Edinburgh* – a move that represents a departure from a tradition of British periodicals, such as the *Critical Review* and the *Gentleman's Magazine*, providing cutting-edge medical news, and in the case of the latter, acting as a 'medical talking-shop'– opened the door for the development of new ways of engaging with medical culture within *Blackwood's*, intended for the reading audiences of the popular nineteenth-century literary magazine.[6]

Edinburgh Medicine and the Founding of the *Edinburgh Review*

The founding of the *Edinburgh* is a tale that quickly turned to legend in the nineteenth century. However, all versions of the tale collude in the inclusion of the surgeon John Thomson in the 'confederacy' that formed to support the first numbers. In a journal entry of 30 September 1802, Francis Horner writes that after the original plan was drawn up between himself, Jeffrey, and Sydney Smith, '[t]he plan was immediately communicated to Murray, Allen, and Hamilton; Brown, Brougham, and the two Thomsons have gradually been made parties'.[7] Thomson was by far the most prolific contributor of medical reviews to the *Edinburgh* in its early years. Today, he is best remembered as the first biographer of William Cullen, and as 'the Old Chairmaker' – a persistent innovator, or, from his opponent's perspective, a radical usurper of the conservative medical faculty at the University of Edinburgh.[8] He was responsible for the creation of a Regius professorship of military surgery in 1806 and the establishment of a separate chair of general pathology in 1831 (to commence in 1832). Duncan, junior, and his father, Andrew Duncan, senior, were similarly innovative.[9] They campaigned heavily for the establishment of the chair in Medical Jurisprudence and Medical Police at the University of Edinburgh and met with strong opposition from the medical faculty. However, during 'The Ministry of All the Talents' (1806–7), the Edinburgh Whigs 'included the study of medical police as part of their scheme for legal reform', and the Duncans were ultimately successful.[10] The appeal of the new liberal Whig review to such men is unsurprising.

Thomson, in particular, would have been well known to Jeffrey as a fellow member of the Speculative Society and as a founder of the Chemical Society, with which the 'Academy of Physics' was merged in 1800.[11] As Geoffrey Cantor has indicated, the ideology of the Academy of Physics foreshadows that of the *Edinburgh*: '[j]ust as the *Review* was founded as a reaction by a group of young men who were dissatisfied with the state of Scotland, so the Academy came into being some five years earlier owing to a similar discontent on the part of some of its first reviewers'.[12] The purpose of the Academy was 'the investigation of Nature, the laws by which her phenomena are regulated, and the history of opinions concerning these laws', and their primary focus was Newtonian science and Baconian inductive methodology – including its applicability beyond the physical sciences.[13] An increasingly nuanced statement on the progress of medical theory and practice, which very much carried on the tradition of the Academy of Physics, arises out of Thomson's contributions to the early numbers of the *Edinburgh*.

The emphasis on empirical observation and practice, rather than theory, in British medicine by the end of the eighteenth century is well documented and often associated with the rise of pathological anatomy following the work of Giovanni Battista Morgagni (1682–1771) and Xavier Bichat (1771–1802) and the founding of medical institutions that allowed for large-scale clinical study.[14] In tune with this wider movement, the medical reviews in the *Edinburgh* deprecate any attempt by an author to privilege individual interpretation or speculative theory over and above the careful collection of empirical data. For example, while the practice of eliminating contagion via fumigation with muriatic acid advocated by Guyton de Morveau is generally met with approval, his theories regarding the action of oxygen on the body are mocked.[15] Immediately following the review of Morveau is another by Thomson, in which he praises John Haygarth's presentation of statistical data via tables: 'upon a subject so obscure in its own nature, as the propagation of contagion, we should feel more indebted to the Doctor for an accumulation of new facts, than for any hypothetical explanations, however ingenious'.[16]

This praise for empirical research is tempered, however, in Thomson's review of Heberden the following year, in language reflexive of the attitudes of Dugald Stewart. In the second volume of his *Elements of the Philosophy of the Human Mind* (1814), after noting the current celebration of inductive methodology by physicians, Stewart builds upon Cullen's medical writings by declaring the futility of experience without some guiding noseological theory: 'without a peculiar sagacity and discrimination in marking, not only the resembling, but the characteristical features of disorders, classed under the same technical name, his practice cannot, with propriety, be said to be guided by any one rational principle of decision, but merely by blind and random conjecture'.[17] Along these lines, Thomson distinguishes between 'true' and 'false' experience in guiding medical practice:

> The former supposes, for its attainment, an historical knowledge of its object, a capacity for observation, and genius to draw proper conclusions; whilst the latter consists only in following blind routine, without reason, and without reflection: in this respect, the enlightened physician is distinguished from the ignorant pretender; and the rational empiric from the mischief-working, contemptible quack.[18]

Serving as an entry point into Thomson's critique of the lack of system in Heberden's treatise, this introductory section also speaks to the wider ideology of the first numbers of the *Edinburgh Review*.

As numerous critics have argued, one of the great innovations of the *Edinburgh Review* was the professionalisation of literary criticism. Contributors were remunerated handsomely, casting Constable as 'enlightened patron' rather than 'tradesman' and transforming the nineteenth-century periodical press into 'a functional equivalent of the cultural authority of Enlightenment philosophers'.[19] As such,

The *Edinburgh Review* opened a new public domain of literary and scientific culture, which it defined in professional, judicial terms as a disciplinary court of judgment and evaluation rather than a marketplace of information and opinion.[20]

In the opening number, the 'Advertisement' famously announces that the review will 'be distinguished, rather for the selection, than for the number, of its articles', and, by their judicious selection, the *Edinburgh Review*, and Jeffrey most particularly, worked to cultivate a reading public defined by shared, enlightened good taste.[21] Taste, rather than originality, took primacy in this post-Enlightenment aesthetics, wherein 'taste' signalled 'a communal organization in which the individual confirms selfhood through similarities'.[22] The arbiters of taste were, of course, the reviewers, and as Mark Schoenfield has argued, through their insistent portrayal of the *Edinburgh* as objective and professional, the modern 'fact' was begotten. However, '[t]his "fact" was not an observable phenomenon, but a theoretical construction based on the accumulation of numerical data and the reiteration of observed phenomenon in persuasively objective narratives'.[23] Similarly, physicians and surgeons such as Thomson solidified professional identity through rhetorical appeals to empirical, scientific practice and enlightened judgement and evaluation.

However, the veil of objective, professional authority at times does wear thin. Thomson aims what is perhaps his most trenchant attack at the figurehead of the medical establishment at the University of Edinburgh, Dr Alexander Monro, *tertius* (1773–1859). Thomson's review of Monro's *Observations on Crural Hernia* (1803) opens by highlighting the grand expectations aroused by Monro's professional eminence and the disappointment that followed perusal of his work. A prime motivation for Thomson to contribute to the *Edinburgh* was most probably self-promotion within the medical marketplace; throughout his career he fought to separate the teaching of surgery from anatomy and to establish a separate professorship of surgery in Edinburgh. In 1777 the Royal College of Surgeons had petitioned the Town Council to establish a separate chair of surgery at the University, but instead Monro, *secundus*, was given the extended title of 'Professor of Medicine, Anatomy, and Surgery', subsequently inherited by his son.[24] Thomson began to give extramural lecturers on surgery in 1800, following his appointment as a surgeon-in-ordinary at the Royal Infirmary; according to his first biographer, his son William Thomson, he was the first person in Edinburgh to systematically cover this topic.[25] In October 1803, when this article was published, Thomson was strategically positioning himself to obtain a professorship of surgery in Edinburgh. His ambition would come to fruition in 1804, not at the University but at the Royal College of Surgeons.[26] One of Thomson's primary criticisms of Monro in the article is the latter's lack of practical experience as a surgeon: 'without having observed the parts in their diseased state (and not in bottles), and often have [sic] watched the skilful surgeon in his operation, and having also practised with his own hands, most erroneous ideas may be entertained'.[27] Hernia was an area of specialty for Thomson (he is, in fact, cited in Monro's treatise), and in this article he carries on from a previous contribution to the *Edinburgh* on hernia in providing details of his own surgical practices.[28] His critique of medical theory is also continued from past reviews, as he accuses Monro's treatise, in common with other medical works, of exhibiting

> that jealous partiality with which an author magnifies any little original remark or hint of a theory into a doctrine of disproportionate magnitude, and dwells upon it with a degree of complacency and copiousness, which he is often obliged to compensate, by retrenching some of the most important parts of the subject.[29]

Perhaps even more damningly, Thomson identifies a rhetoric of the 'curious' in Monro's text – more common in eighteenth-century medical texts, but increasingly viewed as unscientific in the nineteenth century – declaring it to evince 'the wanderings of a mind led astray after curious and strange things, without any sober impression of what is truly useful and important'.[30]

The venomous nature of such critiques did not escape the notice of the medical profession in Edinburgh. In a pamphlet entitled *The Beauties of the Edinburgh Review, alias the Stinkpot of Literature* (1807), the surgeon John Ring (*bap.* 1752–d. 1821), without naming Thomson, criticises his review of Dr Robert Jackson's *Remarks on the Constitution of the Medical Department of the British Army* (1803) for evidencing the 'calumny and detraction' of the *Edinburgh Review* – its self-promotion in the literary marketplace through entertaining defamation.[31] Ring also cites Duncan's 1804 review of Thomas

Thomson's *A System of Chemistry* as exposing the 'jealous and self-interested' agendas of the *Edinburgh's* medical contributors.[32] Duncan is also not named, but Ring cites the editor of the *Anti-Jacobin Review* as remarking that 'Dr. Thompson [sic] has ascertained who this critic is; and that his conduct is the more illiberal, as he is a rival who is endeavouring to lessen Dr. Thompson's [sic] class of pupils, in order to augment his own.' While 'this critic' is also said to be 'the same who vents his spleen in the Edinburgh Medical and Surgical Journal' and a known 'understrapper' to Jeffrey, it remains unclear whether Thomson has correctly identified Duncan, since he does not appear to have been an active extramural or university lecturer at this point.[33] Regardless, it is clear from Ring's pamphlet that the critical authority of the *Edinburgh Review* was being undermined by the palpable self-interest of many of its medical articles. Writing in 1814, the physician Joseph Adams reflects that

> the manner in which medicine was treated in the early numbers, produced a very general disgust among the most respectable part of the faculty. My late friend, Dr. David Pitcairn, on my first return to England, recommended the Edinburgh Review to my perusal, regretting at the same time, that the medical articles did it no credit.[34]

According to Henry Cockburn, Thomson himself 'left the Review from offense, in its infancy'.[35] While the nature of this offense is unknown, Adams notes that an 'eminent physician' informed him 'that the managers had determined to omit noticing any such [medical] publications, as they could not depend on the candour of any one to review them'.[36] Duncan's *Edinburgh Medical and Surgical Journal* instead provided a comparatively more 'polite and dispassionate' periodical context in which to notice the latest medical publications, and it included contributions from medical writers across the political spectrum, while often providing a platform for Duncan's own reforming causes, including his promotion of the rising field of medical jurisprudence.[37]

As Porter has noted, in the nineteenth century 'the medical press was a prime medium for the attainment of greater collective professional self-consciousness and identity'.[38] The *Edinburgh Medical and Surgical Journal*, in particular, built upon its literary cousin's rhetoric of professional critical authority. Its 'Advertisement' echoes that of the *Edinburgh* in declaring the editors' intended selectivity. They announce that, in selecting which texts to review in the 'Critical Analysis' section, 'the Editors will be chiefly regulated by the importance of the subject, the excellence of the manner in which it is treated, and the rarity or expense of the work; and it is their wish rather to bring into notice real improvements, and to encourage diffident abilities, than to discover imperfections, and to expose errors'.[39] Perhaps the professionalising rhetoric of the *Edinburgh Review* could only be realised if medical contributors redirected medical discourse to a less controversial periodical context. However, physiological and anatomical topics continued to be covered with polemical charge.

Whig Ideology and Medico-Scientific Discourse

Joseph Adams's reflections on the negative reception of many of the early medical articles introduce his pamphlet, *An Illustration of Mr. Hunter's Doctrine, particularly concerning the Life of the Blood, in Answer to the Edinburgh Review of Mr. Abernethy's Lectures* (1814), which, according to the advertisement, was printed in order to be bound within copies of the review of John Abernethy's lectures. The review was written by John Gordon (1786–1818), an extramural lecturer in physiology who, like his mentor John Thomson, was 'almost certainly a Whig'.[40] In his review Gordon builds upon the physiological teachings of the surgeon, Whig politician and historian John Allen, a key ideologue of the *Edinburgh* and an early influence on several of its contributors.[41]

Allen is said 'to have lived two quite discrete lives': as an extramural lecturer in physiology in Edinburgh until 1802, and then as an esteemed member of the Holland House set, 'that early nineteenth-century centre of Whig politics'.[42] L. S. Jacyna has persuasively argued that a common thread runs between his physiological and social theories:

> In his 1790 dissertation to the Royal Medical Society he sought to explicate the workings of the human mind without any reference to an immaterial principle. In his lectures on physiology he constructed an account of vitality which dispensed with any form of superadded vital principle as the condition of life and organization. In his political writings, he propounded a naturalistic concept of monarchy which denied that any divine efflation was mingled with the corporeal reality of the king.[43]

Allen's 'Lectures on Animal Oeconomy' (1794–1802) were the first lectures wholly dedicated to an emerging, more systematic 'scientific' physiology to be delivered in Edinburgh. According to Jacyna, in these lectures he forwarded 'a view of the body as de-centralized but coherent', emphasising the chemical 'self-regulating mechanisms' of the animal economy rather than the nervous system.[44] This was a significant deviation from the nervous physiology of Cullen, with its emphasis on the nervous system as the 'central integrating organ'.[45] While noting that Allen himself does not make the connection to Whig politics explicit, Jacyna argues that 'Allen's deposition of the brain and nerves from the pre-eminent place they had occupied in earlier Scottish physiology can now be seen more clearly as an attempt to demonstrate the redundancy of central control.'[46] Among those who are listed as attending his lectures are Gordon and Thomson, along with Francis Horner (1778–1817), Thomas Brown (1778–1820) and Henry Reeve (1780–1814) – all contributors to the *Edinburgh*.[47] Schoenfield has noted the influence of Allen's physiological reasoning on Horner's political economy as exposed in the *Edinburgh* – 'the continuity between the biological and the economic' and his emphasis on 'economics as a material science'.[48] Within the medical marketplace, however, it was Gordon that carried on Allen's legacy after his departure for Holland House (necessitated by the unwelcome reception of his politics in Edinburgh). Daniel Ellis, Gordon's biographer, notes that his decision to offer a separate series of extramural lectures on physiology in 1813, previously taught in conjunction with anatomy, was influenced by the success of Allen's lectures, which 'excited greater interest among the medical students of this school, than any given at that period, either within or without the walls of the University'.[49]

Gordon's motivations for contributing to the *Edinburgh* were clearly, in part, a self-promotional move by an aspiring extramural lecturer striving to get ahead in a fiercely competitive marketplace in which medical students might choose between university lecturers, such as Monro, *tertius* and Duncan, senior, and extramural teachers, like Gordon, Thomson, and even Robert Knox. Contributing to periodicals, even quasi-anonymously, could be advantageous to men of science in developing 'their reputations among the cultural élite': Gordon, for example, was widely considered to be the contributor of the anti-phrenological *Edinburgh* article that famously brought Spurzheim to Scotland to defend his and Gall's new science of the mind, although neither Gordon nor his biographer ever confirmed this attribution.[50] Conversely, anonymous contribution to popular periodicals could also provide a certain freedom from culpability in which, particularly in the case of the *Edinburgh*, the individual might be subsumed within the collective, authoritative 'we' carefully cultivated by Jeffrey.[51]

It is from this collective, authoritative stance that Gordon precedes the better-known surgeon William Lawrence (1783–1867) in attacking Abernethy's lectures on the vital principle. The review is unremittingly harsh, referring to the lectures as 'a collection of bad arguments, in defence of one of the most untenable speculations in physiology; interspersed with not a little bombast about genius, and electricity, and Sir Isaac Newton'.[52] In his vitriolic reaction against any form of speculation, Gordon joins in the chorus of past articles in the *Edinburgh*, which set out the proper methodology and domain of both the physical and mental sciences. Perhaps most poignantly, in a review of Heberden's *Commentaries on the History and Cure of Diseases* (1802), Thomson declares: 'The questions concerning vitality bear the same relation to the study of physiology, and the practice of medicine, as the metaphysical discussions concerning the materiality, or immateriality of the soul, to the phenomena of mind.'[53] Further, physiological reasoning, which Gordon presents as a more plausible alternative to Abernethy's vital principle, is in tune with Allen's influential teachings. Concerning secretion, Gordon writes:

> Although, however, it is yet to be ascertained, to what diversity of chemical influence the blood is subject, in the different organs of the body, we see no reason whatever to doubt, that its conversions are accomplished solely by the operation of those affinities which regulate chemical combination among the particles of matter in general. We are aware, that many sensible persons have imagined, that there is something in living bodies which controls the usual chemical affinities, and forces the elements of these bodies into combinations altogether different from what such affinities would produce; but we own we have often been surprised at the sort of reasoning employed in support of this theory.[54]

According to Jacyna, the root of Allen's radical physiology was his denial of the need for a super-attending vital principle in controlling chemical affinities. Gordon's published lectures on physiology collude with his statements in the *Edinburgh*.[55]

Unsurprisingly, *Blackwood's* (along with the *Quarterly Review*) would take the opposite side of the debate surrounding the vital principle.[56] A later Blackwoodian review of Sir Benjamin Brodie's 'Introductory Lecture' to the Royal College of Surgeons in May 1820 praises Brodie for his attempt to 'prove that the laws which govern life differ from those "which govern the changes of inorganic matter"'.[57] Many of the medical authors who contributed to *Blackwood's* were proponents of the vital principle (and also devoted Tories), such as W. P. Alison, who, unhindered by the complications of political non-conformity (and with familial connections to the Gregory dynasty), went on to hold Cullen's esteemed chair of the practice of medicine at the University of Edinburgh.[58] However, the review of Brodie stands out as relatively atypical in *Blackwood's* in the early 1820s, for its exclusive focus on physiological subject matter and for its lack of obvious literary extrapolation. One of the only comparable articles is D. M. Moir's 'Letter Relative to the Late Dr Gordon' in December 1819. Without discussing Gordon's particular opinions regarding the vital principle, Moir praises the systematic methodology he employs to discover '[t]he laws of organic life, and the wonderful processes by which nature carries on the functions of vitality'.[59] Medical texts are rarely reviewed in *Blackwood's*, and appear to be selected for their cross-referential literary potential (as is the case for Wilson's reviews of medical texts discussed in the introduction above). As such, a neat comparison of the ideological underpinnings of reviews of medical texts and the physiological theories forwarded or critiqued in the *Edinburgh* and *Blackwood's* is not possible. Rather, we must look more broadly to the ways that the magazine engaged with medical subject matter through its 'innovative mixture of literary forms and discourses'.[60]

In their edited volume on science in nineteenth-century periodicals, Gowan Dawson, Richard Noakes, and Jonathan R. Topham argue that '[t]he breakdown of the ideal of a bourgeois public sphere and the developing sense of distinct literary and scientific spheres, was, if anything, more evident in the monthly magazines'. However, they cite the founding of *Blackwood's* as the moment in which a new type of 'self-consciously literary' magazine was born, which discarded the categorisation of articles previously typical of British monthly magazines.[61] As such, medical themes and representations are diffused throughout the magazine. Imaginative and discursive writings engage with contemporary medicine in a range of ways, medical reviews take on a more literary form, and 'reports of advances in medical – or more particularly, coroner's – science' appear in the *Noctes* dialogues.[62] As the following chapter will argue, even the magazine's infamous 'tales of terror' may be read as hybrid medico-literary texts, evolved from the type of popular medical material previously published in monthly magazines. Their Gothic intensification of the embodied first-person singular mode characteristic of *Blackwood's* critical discourse expresses a striking opposition to the disembodied, authoritative, and perhaps even medico-scientific collective discourse of the *Edinburgh*.

Notes

1. [Francis Jeffrey and Andrew Duncan, jr.], 'Willan and others on Vaccination', *ER*, 9 (October 1806), 32–66 (p. 32).
2. Porter, 'Lay Medical Knowledge in the Eighteenth Century', p. 142.
3. Dawson, Noakes, and Topham, 'Introduction', in Cantor et al. (eds), *Science in the Nineteenth-Century Periodical*, p. 4 (on the *Edinburgh Review*, see p. 11).
4. On the *Edinburgh Medical and Surgical Journal*, see Comrie, *History of Scottish Medicine*, vol. 2, pp. 507–11; Loudon and Loudon, 'Medicine, Politics and the Medical Periodical 1800–50', in Bynum, Lock and Porter (eds), *Medical Journals and Medical Knowledge*, pp. 49–69.
5. Hamilton, *The Healers*, p. 196.
6. Rousseau, '"Stung into action . . .": Medicine, Professionalism, and the News', p. 184; Porter, 'Lay Medical Knowledge in the Eighteenth Century', p. 144.
7. As quoted in Clive, *Scotch Reviewers*, p. 196.
8. Jacyna, *Philosophic Whigs*, pp. 78–112.
9. On Duncan, senior, see Chalmers (ed.), *Andrew Duncan Senior: Physician of the Enlightenment*; McCrae, 'Andrew Duncan and the Health of Nations'.
10. Crowther and White, *On Soul and Conscience*, p. 9.
11. Cockburn, *Life of Lord Jeffrey*, vol. 1, p. 54; Cantor, 'The Academy of Physics at Edinburgh 1797–1800', p. 112.
12. Ibid. p. 110. See also Pottinger, *Heirs of the Enlightenment*, p. 4, p. 53.
13. Cantor, 'The Academy of Physics at Edinburgh 1797–1800', p. 111. For the source of this quotation in Cantor's article, see 'Extracts from

the Minutes of the Academy of Physics, vol. i 1797, 1798, 1799', in Welsh, *Account of the Life and Writings of Thomas Brown, M.D.*, pp. 498–9.

14. See Keel, 'The Politics of Health and the Institutionalization of Clinical Practices in Europe in the Second Half of the Eighteenth Century'.

15. [John Thomson], 'Morveau on the Means of Purifying Infected Air', *ER*, 1 (October 1802), 237–43.

16. [John Thomson], 'Dr. Haygarth on Infectious Fevers', *ER*, 1 (October 1802), 245–52 (p. 248).

17. Stewart, *Elements of the Philosophy of the Human Mind*, vol. 2, p. 440. For further on Cullen and philosophy, see Barfoot, 'Philosophy and Method in Cullen's Medical Teaching'.

18. [John Thomson], 'Heberden on the History and Cure of Diseases', *ER*, 1 (January 1803), 466–74 (p. 467). For further on Thomson and Stewart's philosophy, see Jacyna, *Philosophic Whigs*, pp. 135–7.

19. Duncan, *Scott's Shadow*, p. 25.

20. Ibid. p. 26.

21. 'Advertisement', *ER*, 1 (October 1802), 2–3 (p. 2).

22. Schoenfield, *British Periodicals and Romantic Identity*, p. 75.

23. Ibid. p. 52.

24. Jacyna, *Philosophic Whigs*, p. 86.

25. [William Thomson and David Craigie], 'Notice of some of the leading Events in the Life of the late Dr John Thomson, formerly Professor of Surgery to the Royal College of Surgeons, and of Military Surgery in the University of Edinburgh, and more recently Professor of General Pathology in the University', *EMSJ*, 67 (1847), 131–93 (p. 162).

26. Jacyna, *Philosophic Whigs*, p. 89.

27. [John Thomson], 'Dr. Monro on Hernia', *ER*, 3 (October 1803), 136–46 (p. 144).

28. Monro, *Observations on Crural Hernia*, pp. 66–7; [John Thomson], 'Camperi Icones Herniarum', *ER*, 1 (January 1803), 460–6.

29. [Thomson], 'Dr. Monro on Hernia', p. 137.

30. Ibid. p. 140. On the nineteenth-century critique of the curious, see Kennedy, *Revising the Clinic*, pp. 54–5.

31. Ring, *The Beauties of the Edinburgh Review*, p. 1.

32. Ibid. p. 32.

33. Ibid. p. 38. Comrie's list of 'Professors and Lecturers in the Edinburgh Medical School up to 1870' does not include Duncan as a lecturer at this time (*The History of Scottish Medicine*, vol. 2, pp. 628–31).

34. Adams, *An Illustration of Mr. Hunter's Doctrine*, p. 1.

35. Cockburn, *Life of Jeffrey*, p. 143.

36. Adams, *An Illustration of Mr. Hunter's Doctrine*, p. 1.

37. Loudon and Loudon, 'Medicine, Politics and the Medical Periodical 1800–50', in Bynum, Lock and Porter (eds), *Medical Journals and Medical Knowledge*, p. 60. On the promotion of medical jurisprudence in the *Edinburgh Medical and Surgical Journal*, see Crowther and White, *On Soul and Conscience*, pp. 9–10.

38. Porter, 'The Rise of Medical Journalism in Britain to 1800', in Bynum, Lock and Porter (eds), *Medical Journals and Medical Knowledge*, pp. 6–28 (p. 19).

39. 'Advertisement', *EMSJ*, 1 (January 1805), 1–6 (p. 5).

40. Lawrence, 'The Edinburgh Medical School', p. 271.

41. For an overview, see Christie, *The Edinburgh Review and the Literary Culture of Romantic Britain*, pp. 39–58.

42. Jacyna, *Philosophic Whigs*, p. 51.

43. Ibid. p. 76.

44. Ibid. p. 67, p. 71.

45. Ibid. p. 67. For further, see Lawrence, 'The Nervous System and Society in the Scottish Enlightenment'.

46. Jacyna, *Philosophic Whigs*, p. 71.

47. Ibid. p. 190; University of Glasgow Library, Special Collections, MS Gen 1476/A/9250.

48. Schoenfield, *British Periodicals and Romantic Identity*, p. 65.

49. Ellis, *Memoir of the Life and Writings of John Gordon*, p. 108.

50. Dawson, Noakes, and Topham, 'Introduction', in Cantor et al. (eds), *Science in the Nineteenth-Century Periodical*, p. 28. See Ellis, *Memoir of the Life and Writings of John Gordon*, pp. 96–7; van Wyhe, *Phrenology and the Origins of Victorian Scientific Naturalism*, pp. 44–51.

51. On Jeffrey's editorial policy, see Christie, *The Edinburgh Review and the Literary Culture of Romantic Britain*, pp. 39–44.

52. [John Gordon], 'Abernethy on the Vital Principle', *ER*, 23 (September 1814), 384–98 (p. 384).

53. [Thomson], 'Heberden on the History and Cure of Diseases', p. 474.

54. [Gordon], 'Abernethy on the Vital Principle', p. 389. Owsei Temkin has noted the significance of this review as championing 'the chemical explanation of life'. See 'Basic Science, Medicine, and the Romantic Era', p. 98.

55. See Ellis, *Memoir of the Life and Writings of John Gordon*, p. 13; Gordon, *Outlines of Lectures on Physiology*, p. 68.

56. See, for example, [George D'Oyly], 'Abernethy, Lawrence, Morgan, Rennell, on the Theories of Life', *QR*, 22 (July 1819), 1–34. For an overview of the debate on vitality, see Ruston, *Shelley and Vitality*, pp. 1–73.

57. [J. J. Halls], 'Brodie's Introductory Lecture', *BEM*, 8 (January 1821), 419–22 (p. 420).

58. Alison was well known for his advocacy of the 'vital principle' in his lectures at the University of Edinburgh. See L. S. Jacyna, 'Alison, William Pulteney, 1790–1859', *ODNB*, available at http://www.oxforddnb.com/view/article/350 (last accessed 15 June 2016).

59. [D. M. Moir], 'Letter Relative to the Late Dr Gordon', *BEM*, 6 (December 1819), 307–9 (p. 308).

60. Duncan, *Scott's Shadow*, p. 27.

61. Dawson, Noakes, and Topham, 'Introduction', in Cantor et al. (eds), *Science in the Nineteenth-Century Periodical*, p. 12.

62. Parker, *Literary Magazines and British Romanticism*, p. 112.

Chapter 2

The Tale of Terror and the 'Medico-Popular'

Look at the bump, my Lord, upon his head;
Pray feel its brother, on the other side;
And say if, in the range of possibilities,
This poor man here could either rob or steal,
And bear such striking marks of rigid virtue.
Blackwood's Edinburgh Magazine (1821)[1]

The above headpiece for the 'Essays on Cranioscopy', published in *Blackwood's* in August 1821, is cited as the *'Justiciary Records for the year 1996'* and projects the bump-reading rules of phrenology as the court evidence of the future. Combining this determinism with the 'well-known fact' of the malleability of the infant human skull, 'Sir Toby Tickletoby, Bart.' makes a 'modest proposal' to fashion mental caps that 'by repressing the growth of the injurious, and encouraging the expansion of the good affections, would inevitably make all the future generations of Britons to think and act alike for the common welfare'.[2] Further, once phrenologically identified, '[t]he grown up wicked people might be put to death without mercy, for the safety of the good'.[3] Cool, scientific reasoning, bereft of humane feeling, becomes the source of ludicrous horror. This is the article that the *Phrenological Journal and Miscellany* particularly highlights when they declare *Blackwood's* to be 'the most persevering, and, of course, the most absurd of the assailants of phrenology, and enemies of phrenologists'.[4]

The Blackwoodian tale of terror – the genre for which the magazine is most renowned – emerged against a backdrop of medico-scientific progress that was laden with Gothic potential: the development of pathological anatomy, phrenology, and forensic medicine. As the 'champion of the Invisible World' in an age defined by 'utilitarian philosophy and materialism', *Blackwood's* was suspicious of any reductive idiom that privileged progress or utility over aesthetic pleasure, scientific reason over humane feeling, and scepticism over belief.[5] This does not imply that the magazine was 'anti-science', and the present chapter reads the tale of terror as an experimental, dually epistemic and aesthetic literary genre, which evinces a transauthorial attempt in *Blackwood's* to counter the perceived 'opposition between literature, aesthetics, and feeling, on the one hand; and science, utility, and reason, on the other'.[6]

Gianna Pomata defines an 'epistemic genre' as composed of 'kinds of texts that develop in tandem with scientific practices' and are thus 'linked, in the eyes of their authors, to the practice of knowledge-making (however culturally defined)'.[7] Scientific practices relevant to the tale of terror include the writing of case histories, the collection of first-person narratives of unusual subjective experiences, and the introspective and experimental methodologies of Scottish philosophers of mind. I suggest that the genre may be read as a form of hybrid 'medico-popular' writing to be classed alongside non-fiction medical texts such as Robert Macnish's *The Anatomy of Drunkenness* (1827) and *The Philosophy of Sleep* (1830), as well as one of the most canonical 'literary' medical case histories, Thomas De Quincey's *Confessions of an English Opium-Eater* (1822) – first serialised in the *London Magazine* in 1821, but originally intended for publication in *Blackwood's*. The term 'medico-popular' is derived from D. M. Moir's response to *The Anatomy of Drunkenness*, and the first section of this chapter introduces Macnish's first medico-literary project in relation to De Quincey's *Confessions*, before moving on to an examination of the development of the tale of terror in relation to the type of popular medical material previously published in monthly magazines and the case history tradition. The chapter closes by discussing the engagement with the genre by early medical contributors to *Blackwood's*.

The Medico-Popular: Robert Macnish and the English Opium-Eater

In August 1827 Macnish forwarded Moir a copy of his 'Inaugural Essay on Drunkenness'. The two young surgeons had only recently met for the first time in Musselburgh, and in the accompanying letter Macnish notes that although, upon making Moir's acquaintance, 'I forgot to mention that I was a brother <u>lancet</u>, . . . [t]his you will detect at once from the nature of the pamphlet'.[8] This letter begins what would blossom into a lifelong friendship and medico-literary correspondence. Moir responded enthusiastically to Macnish's work, declaring in a subsequent letter that he has 'managed to hit off the subject in such a medico-popular way, as to render it not only instructive to the disciples of Hippocrates, but to Coleridge's "reading public" at large'.[9] His term captures a certain type of Romantic writing that was equally of interest to the 'literary republic', the 'reading public', and the medical profession.[10]

Macnish's text originated as an inaugural dissertation presented before the Faculty of Physicians and Surgeons of Glasgow in 1825. However, according to Moir's posthumous 'Life' of Macnish, published as the first volume of *The Modern Pythagorean; A Series of Tales, Essays, and Sketches* (1838), the essay stood out from the 'mere crambè-recocta common places' typically presented before the Faculty, and the Glasgow publisher William M'Phun 'conceived it might be adapted to the perusal of a wider circle than the one for which it was, originally, altogether intended'.[11] M'Phun's assessment proved true, and by 1834 the text was in its fifth edition.[12] However, its success is attributable to its distinctive literary character, rather than any great degree of medico-scientific novelty. According to Macnish, the two major faults in past writings on drunkenness are, first, their faint and even inaccurate descriptions of the phenomena of drunkenness, and, second, their neglect of the modification of drunkenness according to temperament and inebriating agent.[13] *The Anatomy of Drunkenness* provides florid descriptions of the phenomenological experiences, appearances and behaviours of sanguineous, melancholy, surly, phlegmatic, nervous, and choleric drunkards and distinguishes between the kinds of intoxication produced by wine, ale, spirits, opium, and tobacco.

Thomas Trotter's *An Essay, Medical, Philosophical, and Chemical on Drunkenness and its Effects on the Human Body* (1804) was the first full treatise to treat drunkenness as a medical subject, and Trotter does provide a brief description of the phenomena of drunkenness and the variations of these due to 'natural disposition and temperament'.[14] A comparison of the two authors' descriptions of the first stages of drunkenness reveals the key difference between the texts. Trotter writes:

> The first effects of wine are, an inexpressible tranquility of mind, and liveliness of countenance: the powers of imagination become more vivid, and the flow of spirits more spontaneous and easy, giving birth to wit and humour without hesitation.[15]

While mirroring the same phenomenological sequence, Macnish provides a more 'literary' description, drawing upon vivid figurative language and a nearly poetical rhythm to portray a rich range of sensory transformations:

> First, an unusual serenity prevails over the mind, and the soul of the votary is filled with a placid satisfaction. By degrees he is sensible of a soft and not unmusical humming in his ears, at every pause of the conversation. He seems, to himself, to wear his head lighter than usual upon his shoulders. Then a species of obscurity, thinner than the finest mist, passes before his eyes, and makes him see objects rather indistinctly. The lights begin to dance, and appear double. A gaiety and warmth are felt at the same time about the heart. The imagination is expanded, and filled with a thousand delightful images. He becomes loquacious, and pours forth, in enthusiastic language, the thoughts which are born, as it were, within him.[16]

In his review of the second edition of Macnish's book for *Blackwood's*, Wilson compliments its 'vivid and breathing picture' and includes his own richly poetic descriptions of the horrors of delirium tremens – a phenomenon rife with potential for the tale of terror.[17]

In *The Anatomy of Drunkenness* Macnish responds to a broader valuation of literary men within certain circles of Romantic medico-scientific culture. While he could complain in a letter to Moir that 'doctors . . . are truly a set of dull dogs' and 'perfectly contemptible on every subject not immediately connected with pills and potions', in setting down his views on the origins of nervous diseases in *Hygeia: or, Essays Moral and Medical on the Causes Affecting the Personal State of our Middling and Affluent Classes* (1802–3), Thomas Beddoes sufficiently valued imaginative literature to conclude that his own medical 'project required an inwardness with the ways of the mind that only a creative writer could possess and he called for one to take his place'.[18] Sir Humphrey Davy's nitrous oxide experiments at Beddoes' Pneumatic Institute in Bristol (1799–1802) were in fact performed upon men and women of acclaimed literary merit, and their descriptive reports formed the substance of the experimental data.[19] Macnish includes both Coleridge's and R. L. Edgeworth's phenomenological descriptions in the second edition of *The Anatomy of Drunkenness*.[20] However, the key Romantic medico-literary predecessor for Macnish is De Quincey. Writing to Moir to request permission to dedicate the second edition to 'Delta, Author of "The Legend of Genevieve"', Macnish notes that, should he decline, he will dedicate the book to 'that strange genius the English Opium-Eater'.[21]

De Quincey presents his *Confessions* as a 'useful and instructive' account of 'excess, not yet *recorded*', intended to provide knowledge of the 'fascinating powers of opium', which have been alluded to, but not yet explained by medical writers.[22] Critics have noted the original reception of the *Confessions* as a genuine medical case history,[23] and Macnish cites De Quincey authoritatively on the ability of the body to withstand increasing doses of opium. Like the Opium-eater (and in contrast to Trotter), he also ranks the effects of opium above those of alcohol, declaring '[t]here is more poetry in its visions, more mental aggrandisement, more range of imagination'.[24] Both Macnish and De Quincey aestheticise pathological experience, yoking a Romantic aesthetic of intoxication to epistemic forms of medical writing, and in the opening of the text, as it first appeared in the *London Magazine*, the opium-eater presents his distinctive literary abilities as enhancing the value of his 'case'. Appealing both to a Coleridgean intellectual ideal of subtlety of thought and a Wordsworthian ideal of the 'virtuous poet',[25] as David Higgins notes, De Quincey declares that he has not only sufficient intellect to relate his case, but also an appropriate 'constitution of *moral* faculties, as shall give him an inner eye and power of intuition for the vision and mysteries of our human nature'. He concludes that 'English poets' have had this and 'Scottish Professors' have not.[26]

De Quincey's reference to 'Scottish Professors' alludes to his original intention to publish his 'Opium article' in *Blackwood's*.[27] By December 1820 he had promised an essay on the topic of opium to *Blackwood's*, and in a letter of 19 December he notes it is 'very far advanced'. However, in January 1821 he and William Blackwood quarrelled, and De Quincey soon took the side of the *London Magazine* in the notorious 'cockney school' feud that led to the death of John Scott, editor of the *London*, in a duel with *Blackwood's* representative, Jonathan Christie.[28] Regardless of any ill will towards *Blackwood's*, De Quincey includes a footnote to 'disclaim any allusion to *existing* professors' (i.e. John Wilson) from his general denunciation, and his reference carries forward the magazine's early critique of Common Sense philosophy.[29] A well-known article on Wordsworth in the 'Essays on the Lake-School of Poetry' series in December 1818, for example, opens with the declaration:

> As in this country the investigations of metaphysicians have been directed chiefly towards the laws of intellect and association, and as we have nothing which deserves the name of philosophy founded upon an examination of what human nature internally says of itself . . . we must turn to the poets, if we wish to hear what our literature says upon these subjects.[30]

Lockhart's Peter Morris takes a more extreme stance, concluding that Thomas Brown's and Dugald Stewart's philosophic methods evince 'a very cold and barren way of thinking'.[31] Denouncing the idea of extending 'the empire of science' into the realm of the moral feelings, Morris warns his readers against 'reposing too much confidence in the powers resulting from science' and refers them to Wordsworth – the English poet who 'has better notions than any Scotch metaphysician is likely to have, of the true sources, as well as the true effects, of the knowledge of man'.[32]

The insight into 'the vision and mysteries of our human nature' provided in De Quincey's *Confessions* develops, however, in parallel with a scientific discourse of containment and quantification. As Susan Levin has indicated, the Opium-eater is both a utilitarian, 'a practical being who would analyze everything', and a dreamer 'who submerges himself in the opium experience'.[33] She concludes that in his inability to scientifically analyse his opium dreams, the Opium-eater's confessional text 'becomes a romantic examination of the inadequacy of utilitarian philosophy' that should be read in relation to Shelley's *A Defence of Poetry* and Hazlitt's 'The New School of Reform', in taking 'a stand against the rigidly rational and practical as it dramatizes the justness and power of creative imagination and visionary dreaming'.[34]

The Anatomy of Drunkenness contains a similar tension, but strikes a more confident balance on the side of scientific analysis. Macnish contains his poetic descriptions and aesthetic analysis of the phenomenology of drunkenness within a scientific system that classifies modifications according to temperament and inebriating agent. The Blackwoodian tales of terror also engage with tensions between scientific utility and literary aesthetics, and hence participate in the wider Blackwoodian valuation of '[p]oetry and eloquence' in providing knowledge of human nature inaccessible to 'the empire of science'.[35] However, prior to the advent of this 'medico-popular' genre, the treatment of medical subject matter in the magazine's first incarnation as the *Edinburgh Monthly Magazine* (which lasted for just six months before the launching of *Blackwood's* in October 1817) was remarkably inauspicious.

Magazine Medicine and the Tale of Terror

The first numbers of the *Edinburgh Monthly Magazine* and *Blackwood's* addressed medical subject matter in the same manner as those now stale literary magazines that Blackwood wished to surpass with his new periodical. The 'Medical Reports of Edinburgh' series, introduced in June 1817 and concluded in February 1818, was clearly modelled on a tradition of popular city-specific medical reports, notably sustained for the London context in the *Monthly Magazine* from March 1796 through December 1827. The inclusion of case histories, such as 'Account of the Remarkable Case of Margaret Lyall; Who continued in a State of Sleep nearly Six Weeks', in April 1817, and 'Narrow Escape of the Blind and Deaf Boy, James Mitchell, from Drowning', in June 1817, is likewise typical of contemporary popular magazines.[36] The 'Remarkable Case of Margaret Lyall' was taken directly 'From the Transactions of the Royal Society of Edinburgh' and also published verbatim in the *Scots Magazine* in 1817, carrying on that journal's tradition of publishing 'curious' modern and historical cases.[37] The multifarious aspects of the case of James Mitchell, a boy born blind and deaf, were also well trodden as magazine material. When the London surgeons Sir Astley Cooper (1768–1841) and James Wardrop (1782–1869) attempted to operate to restore Mitchell's sight, the case inspired a resumption of the debates regarding innate versus acquired knowledge via sensory perception begun by William Molyneux in 1688 and carried forward by Locke and the surgeon William Cheselden (1688–1752).[38] Stewart presented an extensive account of his case to the Royal Society in 1812 and also included it in an appendix to the third volume of his *Elements of the Philosophy of the Human Mind* (1827) as fodder against Jeffrey's critique of the possibility of a truly inductive science of the mind.[39] During this period of interest, 'Particulars respecting JAMES MITCHELL, a boy born blind and deaf, and of his visit to London. By James Wardrop' featured in the *Scots Magazine* in March 1813, while 'Particulars respecting James Mitchell, the Boy born Blind and Deaf: by Dugald Stewart. Letter on the same Subject: by Sir James Mackintosh' appeared in June 1814.

The advent of the tale of terror, however, marks a significant shift in the treatment of medical subject matter and the narrative mode in which it is presented. In their anthology *Tales of Terror from Blackwood's Magazine* (1995), Robert Morrison and Chris Baldick provide useful parameters for the genre. Turning to Poe's famous burlesque on 'How to Write a Blackwood Article' (1838), they explain that 'the special intensity noted by Poe is achieved by presenting the recorded "sensations" of a first-person narrator witnessing his own responses to extreme physical and psychological pressures'.[40] Building upon a tradition of sensational crime narratives, peddled to the masses in the form of cheap broadsides and chapbooks, this intense realism was blatantly commercial and intended to attract readers;[41] but it also represents a significant innovation in Gothic form and is 'arguably the single greatest contribution of the Romantic periodicals to the history of short fiction'.[42] As Henry Sucksmith has illustrated, while their Gothic predecessors (and particularly those of the Radcliffean school), generally arouse 'purely romantic terror through vague suggestion', in contrast, the Blackwoodian tales of terror create 'a realistic terror through precision of descriptive detail', which often includes 'a meticulously scientific accuracy'.[43] Morrison and Baldick conclude their definition:

> The usual tone in these stories is one of clinical observation (although without the customary detachment) rather than genteel trepidation, and for the most part the terrors are unflinchingly 'witnessed', not ambiguously evoked: here there are fewer phantoms or rumours of phantoms than actual drowning, suicides, murders, executions, and death agonies.[44]

Their reference to 'clinical observation (although without the customary detachment)', as we will see, is key.

Tim Killick has traced the development of the tale of terror back to the medical case histories appearing in the *Edinburgh Monthly Magazine* and the early numbers of *Blackwood's*, arguing that both the 'potent source material' and the 'tone and structure' of these cases were taken up by the Blackwoodian authors who set the development of the tale of terror in motion.[45] However, in regard to the tale of terror and the case history, Killick neglects an important shift. While each of the case histories included in the *Edinburgh Monthly Magazine* and the early numbers of *Blackwood's* is written in the third person, from the perspective of a philosophical observer – a minister, a surgeon, or an individual collecting material together from recent medical publications – in its classic early form, the tale of terror is written in the first person, from the perspective of the individual who has experienced the physical or mental trauma.[46]

The 'Remarkable Case of Margaret Lyall', in which Lyall's own voice is conspicuously absent, provides a useful contrast. The results of her 'being interrogated respecting her extraordinary state' upon waking for the first time in six weeks are reported in the third person and primarily relate that, with the exception of hearing the voice of a minister who spoke to her on the morning before her return to consciousness, she had no awareness of her mysterious state.[47] A footnote that reports the melancholy denouement of the case – that after her recovery she was found 'hanged by her own hands' – gestures towards her untold story and a potential psychological cause for her protracted sleep and subsequent suicide:

> She is known to have had a strong abhorrence of the idea of her former distress reoccurring; and to have occasionally manifested, especially before her first long sleep, the greatest depression of spirits, and even disgust of life.[48]

Her father's attempts during her protracted sleep 'to rouse her faculties by alarming her fears' of being moved to 'Montrose Infirmary' to be studied by physicians who 'would naturally try every kind of experiment for her recovery' indicates the latent terror of her situation.[49] The terror of a-volitional entrapment in one's own body is, however, explored in vivid detail in later tales of terror such as John

Galt's 'The Buried Alive' in October 1821 and Hogg's 'Some Terrible Letters from Scotland' (published in *The Metropolitan Magazine* in April 1832, but in the Blackwoodian mode), with the additional horror of full mental consciousness.

The first Blackwoodian tale of terror to develop this shift to the first person was Wilson's 'Remarkable Preservation from Death at Sea' in February 1818. The tale is presented as 'a translation of a most interesting letter, addressed to a German gentleman, now resident in Hamburg' who is 'a man of very rare endowments, and the author of several fine Poems'.[50] The letter is the gentleman's attempt to give 'something like a faint shadow' of the miseries he experienced when thrown overboard a ship as a young man, such that 'from it your soul may conceive what I must have suffered'.[51] Accordingly, much of the letter consists of the associative stream of physical sensations and erratic thoughts and feelings that engulf a young man who is thrown overboard from a ship. His extreme experience gains a further dimension of interest when he remembers that he has a 'phial of laundanum' on his person and swallows it, producing at first a pleasurable delirium – a 'mad kind of enjoyment' and a glorious dream vision of having been thrown overboard by a 'mutinous Crew' – which then transitions into a 'cold tremulous sickness' followed by a vision of a 'glorious ghost ship', from which emanates 'the most angelical music that ever breathed from heaven'.[52] Wilson's tale clearly trades upon the fictional author's ability to poetically describe the vivid sensations and imagery prompted by his extreme experience and may be seen as a key precursor to Macnish's and De Quincey's medico-popular writings. A Blackwoodian author attempting to rival Wilson's text two months later, in April 1818, simply dismisses it as 'merely the fiction of some man of poetical genius', marking the onset of competitive writing – with each author attempting to outdo the other, whilst also taking cues from each other's work – that drove forward the early development of the genre.[53]

Just a few months later, Wilson's 'Extracts from Gosschen's Diary' returns to the authoritative framing of the earlier case histories, claiming to be a translation of a Catholic clergyman's journal. However, the tale includes both the sensational first-person narrative of the clergyman, sent to hear a confession in a dungeon, and that of the murderer who forcefully describes the thoughts and feelings that led him, a self-declared 'madman', to kill his lover with pleasure.[54]

Lockhart's tale, 'Christian Wolf. *A True Story from the German*', the following month, is particularly overt regarding the value of such narratives. The tale opens with the declaration:

> The arts of the surgeon and the physician derive their greatest improvements and discoveries from the beds of the sick and the dying. Physiologists draw their purest lights from the hospital and the madhouse. It becomes the psycologist [sic], the moralist, the legislator, to follow the example, and to study with like zeal dungeons and executions, above all courts of justice, the dissecting rooms of guilt.[55]

In dialogue with the medical case histories that at this time were becoming standardised to include post-mortem analyses,[56] the narrator closes his editorial introduction by noting that Wolf's 'blood has already flowed upon the scaffold'.[57] In a narrative predicated upon a court of justice's having declared Wolf guilty of murder and executed him for his crimes, '[i]t is from the height of' not only 'death' but also confirmed guilt 'that one can see and analyse organic dependences and pathological sequences'.[58] However, rather than viewing Wolf with the cool detachment associated with the medical gaze or with the mere 'curiosity' of the casual reader, the narrator declares his intention to educate both 'the heart and the intellect',[59] and exhorts the ideal reader to engage sympathetically with the man, as opposed to viewing him 'as if he were some creature whose blood flowed not with the same pulses, whose passions obeyed not the same law with ours'.[60] The sensational first-person confession included in the tale enables the reader to track these pulses and passions on the pathway to murder.

De Quincey, not without a trace of irony, gestures to a potential post-mortem denouement to his own case history in his 'Appendix' to the *Confessions* in December 1822: he offers his body to 'the gentlemen of Surgeons' Hall' should they 'think that any benefit can redound to their science from inspecting the appearances in the body of an opium-eater'.[61] Galt's 'The Buried Alive' had already depicted a dramatic contrast between a first-person narrative (in this case, of a person in a trance state, first buried alive and then resurrected for anatomical dissection) and the stance of the doctor and students eagerly gazing upon his body. In Galt's tale, some of the students recognise the narrator and 'wish that it had been some other subject', but a series of galvanic experiments and, very nearly, the dissection of his still living body are carried forward, echoing the horrific objectification he has previously experienced at the hands of the crass undertakers, who 'treated what they believed a corpse, with the most appalling ribaldry'.[62] However, the students' pleasure in witnessing the galvanic experiments – the 'admiration' they express for 'the convulsive effect' – mirrors the aesthetic pleasure of the presumed reader of the tale of terror, who, like the lecturer in De Quincey's notorious Blackwoodian essay 'On Murder Considered as One of the Fine Arts' (1827), has a 'taste for violence'.[63]

In De Quincey's essay, after relating a 'remarkable anecdote' in which a student of the Scottish surgeon, William Cumberland Cruikshank, delivers the '*coup de grace*' to an executed criminal, still alive on the anatomy table, the narrator/lecturer posits 'that all the gentlemen in the dissecting-room were amateurs of our class'.[64] His comments appear to have inspired an anonymous essay two months later in the *Monthly Magazine* 'On the Pleasures of "Body-snatching"'. The narrator of the tale is a young student of anatomy with a 'genius' for body-snatching, whose scientific zeal is also accompanied by chilling objectification – an ability to look upon a recent acquaintance as merely 'an anatomical subject' and to explain to a layman who is distressed by the resurrection of a woman's body 'that a dead body was of no sex'.[65] Sir Edward Bruce Hamley's 'A Recent Confession of an Opium-Eater', published in *Blackwood's* in December 1856, inverts this dialectic and depicts the pleasure of the potential anatomical subject who relishes the exposure of dissection. An opium-eater finds himself nearly ensnared by a gang of bodysnatchers in Edinburgh and has a 'refreshing' vision, fantasising that 'all the mighty surgeons and physicians whom the world ever saw' witness Esculapius, 'the great father of physic', cut into his brain, and release 'such a swarm of ideas that the vast hall could not contain them'.[66] The irony is, of course, that the parallel between the confessional genre and anatomical dissection is undercut by the incommensurability of literal dissection and literary revelation.

Alongside such (at times parodic) parallels, medico-scientific objectification also receives a degree of censure in some tales, albeit uncomfortably intermixed with a tacit recognition of the potential pleasures of the medical gaze, and if the tale of terror may be read as offering a potentially poignant perspective from which to critique medico-scientific objectivity, the Gothic aesthetic of the genre may be viewed as a subversion of the developmental trajectory of the medical case history in the nineteenth century. Meegan Kennedy has described how

> the curious discourses common in eighteenth-century case histories – exoticizing, sentimental, sensational, Gothic – were repudiated in favor of a clinical realist discourse that promised to record observations with more objectivity, accuracy, precision, and reliability. The clinical case history deploys all these elements in order to authorize its ideology of objectivity; its aesthetic, a mechanical observation marked by the absent presence of the physician and communicated through a realist discourse; and its product, the medical fact.[67]

While more realistic than its Gothic predecessors, the tale of terror certainly eschews 'mechanical observation' and instead sets up a dialectic between the empirical narrator's sensational relation of the events and the putatively authoritative medico-scientific narrative. For example, a footnote from the 'Editor' in 'Narrative of a Fatal Event' indicates the potential unreliability of the emotive narrator. The tale is written from the perspective of a guilt-ridden man, who many years earlier was unable to save a drowning friend due to a 'horror . . . acquired when a boy, from an exaggerated description of the danger of the convulsive grasp of a person drowning'.[68] At a critical point he claims to have seen an uncanny vision of his friend, still alive beneath the water and seated 'upright', and the 'Editor' indicates that the 'appearance might arise from the refraction of the agitated water, as well as from the excited imagination of the narrator'.[69] This sceptical dynamic would reach its forte in Hogg's *The Private Memoirs and Confessions of a Justified Sinner* (1824). However, it is also present in the 'Appendix' to De Quincey's *Confessions*, in which the opium-eater worries about the potential for others to perceive his reporting of his case as unreliable. He admits that he has erroneously led the reader to believe that he has 'wholly renounced the use of Opium', and one of his reasons for doing so, he claims, is 'because the very act of deliberately recording such a state of suffering necessarily presumes in the recorder a power of surveying his own case as a cool spectator, which it would be inconsistent to suppose in any person speaking from the station of an actual sufferer'.[70]

As Peter Logan has argued, in this passage De Quincey is working 'to negotiate the paradox' of what Logan terms the 'nervous narrative', since 'any early-nineteenth-century narrative of a personal history filled with painful sensations raises questions about the narrator's present clarity of mind'.[71]

In featuring the first-person narratives of actual sufferers, the tale of terror might then be read as a form of nineteenth-century 'autopathography' which counters the authority and objectification of the medical case history and provides a story of human suffering.[72] De Quincey's *Confessions* has been read as '*anti*-medical',[73] and follows on from a 'Medical Article' series in the *London Magazine*, written from the perspective of a physician wishing to deliver useful knowledge, that only lasted through their first four numbers.[74] Charles Lamb's 'Confessions of a Drunkard' in August 1822, and Bryan Waller Procter's 'The Memoir of a Hypochondriac' in September and October 1822, carried forward De Quincey's example. Even the *Monthly Magazine* discontinued printing physicians' medical reports by December 1827 and instead featured tales from the patient perspective, such as 'On Hypochondriasis' (July 1826) and 'Recollections of a Night of Fever' (May 1829). However, we might also view the tale of terror as reflecting the value placed on first-person experience in the empirical project of post-Enlightenment medicine. As we will see in Chapter 4, the publication of Warren's *Passages from the Diary of a Late Physician* in 1830 shows the medical profession itself taking on this narrative mode, with the late physician claiming that 'experience is the only substratum of real knowledge'.[75] Shortly afterwards the *Monthly Magazine* followed suit with the medico-popular series 'Experiences of a Surgeon', which ran through five numbers in 1835.

Such potential tensions and convergences between medico-scientific developments, the tale of terror, and Blackwoodian Romanticism more broadly feature in the writings of early medical contributors to the magazine. In the remainder of this chapter, I turn to three medical figures – John Howison, William Dunlop, and Robert Macnish – each of whom engaged with the tale of terror in some way. Their work opens up an alternative narrative of Scottish medicine in the early nineteenth century: one that acknowledges the often-cited importance of empirical scientific practices in post-Enlightenment Edinburgh medicine, but also highlights close engagement with the aesthetics of literary Romanticism. As we will see, synergistic potentials are realised, while ideological conflicts between Blackwoodian Romanticism and Scottish medicine also come to light.

John Howison, the Quantitative Tale of Terror, and Medical Travel Writing

Between May 1821 and July 1822, the 'main contributor of fiction' to *Blackwood's* was a surgeon with a particular proclivity for both the tale of terror and, as Anthony Jarrells has recently indicated, the 'regional tale'.[76] John Howison was born in Edinburgh, the son of a financial writer, and he was a medical student at the University of Edinburgh from 1812 to 1816. However, rather than taking his MD, from 1818 to 1820 he travelled to Ontario and Quebec, practising medicine and gathering materials for his first travel book, *Sketches of Upper Canada, Domestic, Local, and Characteristic* (1821). As Bonnie Shannon McMullen indicates, before returning to Britain after his Canadian adventures, Howison, 'having accepted an appointment as a surgeon with the East India Company . . . seems to spend his last months of freedom exploring the West Indies'.[77] During the short period that he was in Edinburgh and in London before finally departing for Bombay, he became a contributor to *Blackwood's*, most probably through the connections of his elder brother William, who was a frequent contributor.

Howison's tale 'Adventure in Havana', which appeared in *Blackwood's* in June 1821, places a man avowedly of the 'medical profession' at the heart of a multiplicitous colonial tale of terror.[78] McMullen reads this tale in relation to the chapter on 'The City of Havana' in Howison's *Foreign Scenes and Travelling Recreations* (1825), and views his exploration of the devastating death toll of the yellow fever metaphorically, as indicative of the 'moral infection' of an economic system based on mercantile greed and the slave trade.[79] The tale also clearly recycles material from previous Blackwoodian tales of terror, including 'Remarkable Preservation from Death at Sea' and 'Narrative of a Fatal Event'. The opening relates the protagonist's feverish dream vision, in which he loses 'all sense of external objects' and believes he has fallen overboard, only to be surrounded by 'floating bodies of dead seamen tied upon planks'. At the climax of the dream a corpse that he has attempted to grasp and float upon comes to life, utters a 'horrible shout', and attempts to drag him to the depths.[80] The style of Howison's narrative was sufficiently similar to previous tales of terror to make Moir ponder, in a letter to Blackwood, 'the Adventure in Havana is a piece of powerful conception, and forcible writing: is it not by the [same author as] "Narrative of a fatal evident [sic]" and "The Hospital Scene" and "Gosschen's Diary"?'[81] The key difference is that in Howison's tale, following his own traumatic experience (which gestures towards depths of meaning outwith the reach of the 'empire of science'), the medical narrator becomes a collector of similar, albeit less subjectively aestheticised, narratives. The remainder of the tale is devoted to the narratives of three other dying men, also infected with yellow fever, all of whom are entrapped within the same 'private hospital' as the narrator.[82]

In shifting the tale of terror from singularity to multiplicity, Howison brings the genre into closer engagement with contemporary medical trends. With the rise of a 'critical approach' in eighteenth- and early nineteenth-century medicine, mass observation and quantifying methods, which required the gathering of numerous cases, became increasingly valued.[83] Within medical periodicals there was a 'gradual reduction in dependence on single case reports and a growth in the publication of ever larger case series', assisted by the opportunities for mass observation generated by the eighteenth-century British hospital movement, military medicine and the work of the East India Company.[84] This shift was particularly associated with Edinburgh medicine – the teachings of Cullen, the sceptical and empirical philosophy of Hume, its revision by Reid and Stewart, and the reaffirmation of inductive methods by their medical followers.

Howison devoted a substantial portion of the dissertation he presented to the Royal Medical Society in the 1816–17 term, 'On the Remote Causes of Death', to the sheer difficulty of tracing the causal chain of the wide range of interactive 'external agents' that progressively lead to death and decay in each individual.[85] However, in tune with the quantitative methods favoured in Edinburgh medicine, he explains that 'we may, if particular phenomena be present in the one class of persons, and absent in the other, reasonably ascribe such to the operation of those agents which were known to act in the one case, and not in the other'.[86] One may apply this reasoning to 'Adventure in Havana'.

The narratives amassed by the medical narrator come from three men with distinctive characters and personal histories. The first is an ill-tempered and vengeful smuggler from Orkney, with a nearly pathological attachment to his homeland; the second, a doting father and merchant from Baltimore who is only concerned that he does not infect his daughter; and the third, a naïve young man from Philadelphia who has been cheated out of his money and health and longs only to return to his fiancée in America. Amongst their differences, however, all three hold in common an intense, emotive reaction to the knowledge that they are dying and are to be separated from their loved ones. In contrast, during the crisis of his own illness the medical narrator reflects:

> I knew that I was attacked by the yellow fever, and I also knew that few of my age or temperament ever recovered from it. I was a friendless stranger in a foreign land. But the thoughts of this did not depress me.[87]

He is the only man of the group to survive the fever, inviting the quantitatively minded reader to consider the possible reasons. In his medical dissertation Howison placed particular emphasis on 'mental agents', declaring that '[e]very idea, every emotion, produces a corresponding change in the state of the body' and noting 'they sometimes affect the frame much more vehemently, than external causes'.[88] This, along with his preoccupation throughout his writings with the potentially deleterious consequences when 'some deep emotion, or particular train of ideas takes possession of [the mind], to the exclusion of all others', suggests that the other men's emotional states, while providing excellent source material for a tale of terror, may have prevented their recoveries.[89] Collectively, the narratives echo Howison's description of the pathological foreign adventurer in *Foreign Scenes and Travelling Recreations*, who, disillusioned with his adventure, 'becomes hypochondriac, sickens, and dies, and is carried to his solitary grave by strangers and hirelings'.[90] In Howison's hands the tale of terror maintains its sensational subjective depths, with the added exoticism of a foreign clime of tropical disease and mercantile corruption, while also opening up further empirical possibilities for the young surgeon.

Many of Howison's subsequent Blackwoodian tales, such as 'The Florida Pirate' and 'Adventures in the North-West Territory', as well as his full-length works, which included *Tales of the Colonies* (1830) and *European Colonies, in various parts of the world, viewed in their social, moral, and physical condition* (1834), draw upon the knowledge he gained through his extensive travels. His *Sketches of Upper Canada* was particularly popular, and in turning to travel writing, Howison participated in an established medico-literary tradition.[91] In the eighteenth and early nineteenth centuries, Scottish medical graduates often completed their education with a 'Medical Tour' of continental medical academies, before forging colonial careers as physicians or surgeons in the navy, army or with the East India Company, and those with literary proclivities frequently published accounts of their travels. Smollett's kinsman Dr John Moore (1729–1802), for example, drew on his experiences of the Grand Tour in his capacity as tutor-physician to the Duke of Hamilton and a military surgeon, to become a very popular travel writer.[92]

Within the popular periodical press, one function of medical travel writing was to provide an account of the progress of medicine in other countries – and in Scotland or England for other countries. The *Scots Magazine*, for example, features a series of articles between December 1808 and April 1809 entitled 'Description of Edinburgh: with an Account of the present State of its Medical School', which comprised a series of translated letters from the German physician Johann Peter Frank (1745–1821), who had visited the university while Lecturer of Pathology at Wilna. The letters contain a detailed account of Edinburgh and its society, the history of the university, the medical curriculum, the professors and their lecturing styles, graduation, and key institutions and societies. Frank is particularly generous in his commendation of the students:

> In Edinburgh there prevails a more solid and better tone of Society, and a more genuine zeal for knowledge among the studious youth. They have an opportunity of enjoying the conversation of the Professors. What particularly augments the ardour for knowledge among the students, is the learned conversations which take place among them.[93]

Frank's letters conclude in May 1809 with an 'Account of the Town and University of Glasgow'. As with the Edinburgh letters, his account is neatly divided into subsections, describing the university and key medical institutions, and written from the stance of an impartial observer (which is only slightly interrupted by the discomfort of his journey to Glasgow and a particularly offensive inn).

Characteristically, *Blackwood's* turns this form of medical writing on its head through the medium of prose fiction. In his humorous medico-popular travel tale, 'Vanderbrummer; or, the Spinosist' (December 1821), an account of a Dutch medical student who has completed his studies at Leyden and travels to Britain to finish his education, Howison provides a running commentary on the state of medicine in England and in Edinburgh. However, rather than an impartial observer, 'Vanderbrummer' reflects the stance of the most famous Blackwoodian travel-writer: Lockhart's Dr Peter Morris. As mentioned in the introduction, Francis Hart has described Morris's stance as a 'Romantic cultural observer', evincing the 'shift from the objective to the subjective in romantic travel writing':[94]

> For the reader whose tastes were formed on memoir, diary, and historical romance, the authentication of the cultural observer lay in his closeness to his subject, his partiality for the biases of the milieu he describes or represents. . . . He will need to be sympathetically or antipathetically alive to the 'character' or the spirit of what he sees. A culture – like a personality – can be awakened to life only by a personality.[95]

Vanderbrummer's personality is marked by his metaphysical enthusiasm. From his youth he 'had inclined most towards thought concerning substantive existence, and he often wished to lose all differences of feeling, in the notion of an universal community of being, and relationship with nature'.[96] He is thus delighted when he discovers the writings of Spinoza, which show him how 'by logical deduction' he might prove 'what he wished habitually to feel'.[97] The cultural observer is characterised as a medical theorist, and in post-Enlightenment Scotland, such a characterisation was hardly complementary.

The increasing utilisation of quantitative methods was part of the general reaction against 'theory-based dogma' in British medicine and surgery.[98] While in Germany, Schelling could apply Kant's transcendental metaphysics in his attempt to formulate an *a priori* philosophical science of medicine, in Scotland Cullen's Baconian inductive approach predominated, with authorities such as John Gregory warning against the dangers of not only theory but also 'over-heated imaginations' in their published works.[99] This was also a dominant discourse within medical societies and in journals. John Thomson, in his 1808 Royal Medical Society dissertation, 'Has Theory tended to promote or retard the Science of MEDICINE', denounced the peril of the 'flimsy cob-web theories of the day' that 'steal from the warm ingenious youth, those valuable hours which ought to have been sacrificed to harder and more useful study, while they hold out expectations which can never be realized'.[100] Such statements were tempered by those who perceived the theoretical utility of Common Sense philosophy in medicine. However, this particular utilisation of 'theory' was still associated with inductive, *a posteriori* reasoning and was contrasted with the 'false' theoretical systems of the past, as '[t]he history of medicine, and the annals of the rise and decline of successive theories, show how deficient were their authors in all the requisites of accurate observation, sound reasoning, and legitimate deduction'.[101]

Vanderbrummer, as a 'Spinosist', is a medical theorist on overdrive. As Stuart Hampshire explains, the Dutch philosopher Baruch Spinoza (1632–77) was the champion of *a priori* philosophy, and 'no other philosopher has ever insisted more uncompromisingly that all problems, whether metaphysical, moral or scientific, must be formulated and solved as purely intellectual problems, as if they were theorems in geometry'.[102] However, Antonio Damasio has also recently brought attention to Spinoza's rooting of all rational thought in the emotive body – an idea currently receiving new attention in contemporary neuroscience.[103] Appropriately, then, Vanderbrummer's metaphysical system comes under threat on his journey, first by his experience of seasickness:

> Every thing then appeared hateful and distorted, and he thought with contempt and aversion on the pursuits he had formerly delighted in. All his opinions seemed erroneous and unfounded; and he began to despise himself and his fellow-creatures, as beings who were incapable of resisting causes of pain, and unable to evade the degrading influences of adventitious circumstances.[104]

His week in England with Dr L—, 'a short, stout, corpulent man, bold and assuming in his manners, and impatient of contradiction, though very liberal in using it towards others', further frustrates his innate philosophical beliefs, as he 'could not help feeling a degradation in believing that the lowest, stupidest, and basest individuals were entirely of the same stuff as himself; for hitherto he had not been displeased to own an alliance with inanimate nature'.[105] Amongst other charming habits, including a contemptuous bedside manner, Dr L— performs 'experiments to shew how small a quantity of nutriment was sufficient for the support of the animal economy' and, in an ironic perversion of Vanderbrummer's philosophy, argues that '[a]ll articles are equally nourishing, and equally convertible into chyle', serving up 'soup made from the sawings of beech timber' for his dinner.[106]

Happily, Vanderbrummer soon meets another medical companion, Dr Winter, who is of a more congenial turn of mind. In regard to English medicine, Winter remarks that 'medical science is at a low ebb in this country. There is no such thing as theory now', and he suggests that Vanderbrummer travel to Edinburgh, where 'the science of medicine is taught in all its purity'.[107] However, his tour of the Edinburgh medical school, under the guide of a 'Dr Practic', proves disappointing (particularly in contrast to Frank's high praise in the *Scots Magazine*). Vanderbrummer is shocked by the 'levity of deportment which the students exhibited' in the lecture hall, and when he attempts to discover 'what theory of life was then most prevalent among Scotch physicians', the only response he receives is from a student who insists: 'I know nothing about the matter. – I expect to learn all these things from my *grinder*.'[108] Similarly, when Vanderbrummer attends a student dissertation presentation and debate at the Royal Medical Society, he finds that '[a]ll that was advanced by the disputants on either side of the question, had evidently been gleaned from books; and he who remembered most, enjoyed the reputation of speaking best'.[109]

Vanderbrummer eventually returns to his home in Amsterdam only to become 'again interested in the old chain of arguments which had formerly pleased him at Leyden', despite learning through the course of his travels that his metaphysical theories do not meet the test of experience.[110] However, his harsh observations regarding Edinburgh medical culture subject the opposite extreme – the imitative repetition of facts, with no real mental engagement – to equal criticism. The reproach was not original. In 1808 Thomas Beddoes referred to the Edinburgh medical faculty as a place where 'at once degrees are conferred and lectures systematically read' and complained about the industrial scale of its 'triennial manufactory'. In March 1821, in a humorous letter under the Christopher North pseudonym in *Blackwood's*, William Maginn refers to Edinburgh as a city containing 'a regular vomitory for doctors of medicine'.[111]

In this, the Blackwoodian critique of Edinburgh medicine mirrors the critique of the Edinburgh Whigs. Dr Morris asserts that the Edinburgh Whigs are 'a very disagreeable set of pretenders' whose knowledge is entirely 'derived from the Edinburgh Review itself'.[112] Instead, Morris celebrates singular characters, such as Howison's brother William, musing:

> By what process of circumstances such a mind as his is, should have been formed and nurtured into its present condition, in the midst of the superficial talkers and debaters of Edinburgh, I am greatly at a loss to imagine.[113]

Like Vanderbrummer, William Howison was a theorist – according to Sir Walter Scott, a 'metaphysician full fifty fathom deep' – and his originality lay primarily in his utter disregard for the dominant inductive approach.[114] For example, in 'An Essay on the Arrangement of the Categories', contributed to *Blackwood's* in 1822, he delineates twelve categories, relating 'particular existence to the ideal, or the possible modes of being' and argues that 'those twelve deities, which the ancients reckoned as composing the council of the gods, were representations of the twelve categories'.[115] He subsequently carried this work forward in *The Contest of the Twelve Nations; or, a View of the Different Bases of Human Character and Talent* (1826), which turned phrenological empiricism on its head by appealing to both empirical observation *and* ideal possibilities in delineating the, again, twelve generic characters of man, each of which is dominated by a 'triad' of three phrenological organs, which are 'only a different application of the same abstract principle'.[116] In reviewing the text, the *Phrenological Journal* pronounces upon the evident pathology of the author, declaring:

> In our last Number we noticed the case of an individual in whom all intellectual ideas were invariably associated with colours: we have a strong impression that, in the author of the present work, the organs of Form and Size preponderate to excess, and invest his general conceptions with

the attributes of magnitude and form. He manifests a tendency to view the phenomena of the whole world, physical, moral, and intellectual, with all their relations, through the medium of, or in connexion with, the two faculties now mentioned.[117]

This was exactly the type of distinctive subjectivity celebrated in *Blackwood's*. If Howison viewed the world through 'the organs of Form and Size', Christopher North interpreted the world through his gouty toe, the Ettrick Shepherd through a dizzy haze of whiskey punch and canny superstition, and Dr Morris through his own hobby-horsical obsession with the craniological science. However, while, as Vanderbrummer's tale humorously reveals, this aspect of Blackwoodian ideology was at odds with mainstream Edinburgh medicine, the medical marketplace could also accommodate original characters.

The Aesthetics of Forensic Medicine: 'Tiger' Dunlop in the Medical Lecture Theatre

In November 1823 the *Edinburgh Advertiser* announced:

> Mr. W. Dunlop will deliver a Course of Lectures on Forensic Medicine, on Mondays, Wednesdays and Fridays, at four o'clock in the Clyde Street Hall, during the Winter Term of the Court of Session – commencing on Wednesday, November 19th. Tickets Three Guineas.[118]

The lectures were marketed primarily to the legal profession and were intended to supplement the military surgeon William Dunlop's modest income as a half-pay officer and occasional contributor to *Blackwood's* (under the pseudonym 'Colin Ballantyne').[119] Although he was a privileged son of the 'Dunlops of Dunlop', a reversal in his father's fortunes, caused by the failure of a cotton mill in Rothesay, necessitated that the young man make his own way in the world.[120] He served as a medical officer in Canada in the War of 1812 in 'Blayney's Bloodhounds' (the 89th Foot) and also spent time in India, at first attempting to establish himself as a businessman in Calcutta through family connections, then turning to journalism, and finally embarking on a tiger-hunting adventure on Saugur island that earned him the nickname 'Tiger' Dunlop. An attack of 'jungle fever' brought about his return to Scotland in May 1820. While convalescing on Bute he penned a series of humorous sketches on 'Calcutta' for *Blackwood's*, one of which contains a self-portrait:

> In a corner, stood a strong broad-shouldered, carroty-haired, slovenly, coarse-looking Scotchman, . . . the editor of a Calcutta paper who soon after abandoned his literary career for one as hopeless and less profitable, a wild-goose scheme of clearing the Island of Saugur in the mouth of the Ganges of jungle [sic], where he found aborigines (tigers and alligators) more a match for him than his political opponents, and, as every one expected, he soon lost his health, and is now, I believe, enjoying the fruits of his folly in Scotland.[121]

When he made his way to Edinburgh, he quickly fell back into the society of his early school friends, Wilson and Lockhart, and joined their 'Ambrosianæ' circle. Dunlop's decision to lecture on the topic of forensic medicine may have been informed by the popularity of the subject amongst his Blackwoodian friends.

In the early nineteenth century, forensic medicine formed one half of the burgeoning field of medical jurisprudence, which was one of the most innovative areas of Scottish medicine. Until 1830 the University of Edinburgh was the only UK institution to have a professorial chair dedicated to the field that encompassed both public health, or 'medical police', and forensic medicine. As outlined in Chapter 1, the chair, first held by Andrew Duncan, junior, was linked to progressive politics and the reform of medical education. More broadly, as Catherine Crawford has argued, the field became a focal point for those who 'sought to make the medical art more objective and certain', as it uniquely demonstrated the power and utility of particularly 'scientific' fields of medical enquiry, such as chemistry and pathological anatomy, by emphasising their diagnostic acumen.[122] The burgeoning field also enabled courts of law to become an important arena for the establishment of medical power, as the 'standards of evidence' required within a court of law were deemed 'appropriate to the objective, certain, scientific knowledge that reformers envisaged for medicine in general'.[123]

The two subsequent appointments to the university chair, William Pulteney Alison, who held the chair from 1820 to 1821, and

Robert Christison (1797–1882), who held it from 1821 until 1832, were well-known Tories who lessened the Whiggish associations with the field in Scotland; the work of Christison in his specialty of chemical toxicology, in particular, also brought the forensic component of the field further to the forefront.[124] Christison maintains his fame today as one of the Edinburgh medical men who formed the basis for Conan Doyle's 'Sherlock Holmes', and perhaps unsurprisingly the increased emphasis on forensic medicine, in turn, lent the field a particular popular appeal. As Robert Gooch notes to John Murray, 'the subjects are as interesting as the "Chronicles of the Cannongate [sic]"'.[125]

Blackwood's had a partiality for the subject. A lengthy review, 'Hints for Jurymen', published in June 1823, just a few months before Dunlop's lecture series was announced, praises J. A. Paris and J. S. M. Fonblanque's *Medical Jurisprudence* (1823) for the 'great merit' of being 'a most amusing as well as a most instructive and learned book'.[126] The review's extensive extracts from the text discuss feigned insanity, deafness, blindness, and somnolency, as well as cases of spontaneous combustion, trance, premature burial, unexpected resuscitations, unsuccessful hangings, and murder. While claiming to call attention to the importance of forensic medicine and the need to educate 'jurymen' such that medical evidence may be correctly interpreted, the review is really an exercise in sensationalism, containing just the type of material that tales such as 'The Buried Alive' and 'Le Revenant' exploited.

Heather Worthington has discussed the link between forensic medicine and Blackwoodian fiction at length, focusing upon tales of terror and what she terms 'social fables', such as Wilson's 'The Forgers' (1821) and 'The Expiation' (1830), which contain narratives of crime.[127] She argues that while reconstituting '[t]he individual, who is objectified in the broadsides . . . as subject in the attempt to depict the subjective experience of the criminal', *Blackwood's* short fictions also emphasis the readability of the criminal body and assert a disciplinary authority, at times 'filtering their criminal narratives through the voice of a respectable, often religious or medical, narrator, and by resorting to a third-person narration'.[128] For Worthington this discourse continues to develop through Samuel Warren's *Passages from the Diary of a Late Physician* and culminates in the rise of detective fiction. In the context of contemporary medical culture, however, rather than later literary trajectories, Dunlop's lectures provide additional insight into the strange collusion of sensationalism and disciplinary authority and reveal that, while forensic medicine was associated with the rise of medical authority in the public sphere, medical sensationalism and (in Dunlop's particular case) medical waggishness could still flourish and, indeed, be beneficial to the medical professional.

Beyond his experiences as a military surgeon, the 'Tiger' had no real qualifications to deliver a course on forensic medicine, and an extant partial manuscript copy of his lectures explains his preparations. Dunlop's 'Introductory Lecture' notes his 'good fortune, by the kind indulgence of the learned judge, who presides over our supreme criminal court' in obtaining 'access to the accurate notes taken by his Lordship, on every case tried before him, since he took his seat on the bench'.[129] Accordingly, detailed accounts of a rich range of criminal trials drawing upon medical evidence fill out the bulk of the lectures. Dunlop lists key medical figures in Edinburgh, including 'Dr. Thomson Dr. McIntosh & Dr. John Scott – Staff Surg. Marshall Mr. Liston & Mr. Syme', as supporters of his work, and acknowledges the assistance of 'younger friends in the profession of the law'.[130] Despite his lack of an established reputation in the field, and thanks to the combination of potent source material and his own particular style, Dunlop appears to have been successful. Lockhart's Blackwoodian review of Theodrick Beck's *Elements of Medical Jurisprudence* (1825), which includes 'notes, and an Appendix of Original Cases, and the latest discoveries; by William Dunlop', notes that this 'William Dunlop' is 'the same gentlemen whose excellent lectures on medical jurisprudence attracted so large a share of public attention, last year, here in Edinburgh'.[131] In a later article for *Fraser's*, Maginn recalls the lectures: 'the mixture in which of fun and learning, of law and science, blended with rough jokes, and anecdotes not always of the most prudish nature, will make them live long in the memories of his hearers'.[132]

Like the many literary figures associated with *Blackwood's*, Dunlop developed a signature style and an accompanying persona. As Elizabeth Baigent explains, '[t]he success of Dunlop's writings depended on his conscious cultivation of himself as comic hero, and this also left a legacy of tales and legends of his feats, adventures, and practical jokes which long outlived him'.[133] This 'conscious cultivation'

continued in the medical lecture theatre. In the script of his 'Introductory Lecture', the annotation 'Strunt' appears on eight different
occasions, most often in the side margin at the beginning of a new
section. As the Scots term for 'strut', one may imagine the military
man and larger-than-life humorist holding court, with his imposing
theatricality undercut by humorous asides and ludicrous suggestions.
In discussing a preparation of arsenic known as 'King's Yellow' in a
lecture on poisons, he mentions, 'I have never heard of any instance
of its doing harm except in the case of a country woman who thought
it would be a good substance to colour her cheese with', and while
discussing the 'Dissection of Bodies for Juridical Purposes' he suggests that one might 'take off the head' of a corpse, if unidentified,
and 'carefully preserve it in spirits for the purpose of being identified at some future period by the friends of the deceased'.[134] Practical
information is interlaced with (misogynistic) military bravado: in his
lecture on 'Rape', in discussing the 'discretion and discrimination . . .
necessary in concluding that a woman has been overcome by force,
where neither intimidation nor stupification is alleged', he posits an

> argument against a woman being overcome by force, which was first
> stated to me by a worthy friend of mine, a Naval Officer of high rank
> and long standing in his profession – He said that the muscles of the
> thigh of any one human being were too powerful to be separated the one
> thigh from the other by the force of almost any other human being – and
> as a proof of this he put a silk handkerchief round each of his thighs, and
> giving the ends to two strong midshipmen allowed them to pull with all
> their force, sitting on deck with their feet purchased against each other,
> but without the slightest effect being produced.[135]

Even the most macabre of topics – the wasting corpses of stillborn
babes – loses all gravity in Dunlop's hands. In explaining why one
should be cautious in launching a full-blown investigation when a
dead infant is found, he notes: 'We are told that in France the Police
were caused much trouble from the carelessness of some young
Anatomists who having an oversupply of Fœtuses for the purpose
of dissection were apt to dispose of them overplus [sic] by the easi-
est means, and that too perhaps with suspicious looking gashes in
their body.'[136] In Ireland, he believes a similar problem may surface
as stillborn infants are 'exposed out of doors the night after their
birth as a propitiatory offering to the Fairies or as they call them

the good people and if by any accident a Hog or Dog or Bird of prey should carry it off its parents have the consolation to think that their offspring is in a fair way of figuring as a Hero or Heroine in Fairy-Land'.[137] Dunlop presents himself as the surgeon willing to fire a gun in a sleeping patient's room to prove feigned deafness and as a sidekick to the physician who tortures a man, supposedly in a trance, with 'blisters, electricity, galvanism, showerbaths, pricking with needles, red hot wires, injecting hartshorn up the nose and a series of tortures that might have done credit to the Inquisition', only to use a simple trick to finally expose him.[138] In his hands forensic medicine becomes entertaining, at least if one has a 'taste for violence', and at times even ludicrously theatrical.[139] Displays of scientific acumen are there, but with a heavy dose of waggery.

Following on from his lectures, Dunlop became editor of the second edition of Beck's *Elements of Medical Jurisprudence*, published by John Anderson in London, in partnership with William Blackwood in Edinburgh and Hodges and M'Arthur in Dublin. In a letter to Blackwood in September 1824, Dunlop is notably blasé regarding the work. He writes:

> I had no interest in the med. work that Anderson wrote you about further than as being editor I should like to see it prosper as I have no doubt it will as it is by far the best work on the subject in ours or I think any other language my notes & preface are of very little consequence further than giving it an english form & an english name but I am quite sure it will sell.[140]

In his *Blackwood's* review, 'Beck and Dunlop on Medical Jurisprudence', Lockhart was less sanguine regarding Dunlop's contribution, praising the 'picturesque anecdotes' contained in his additional notes for throwing 'new and important light on the topics under discussion, so as to render them extremely valuable to professional readers', while 'presented in a style so natural and original, that, we are quite sure, they must add greatly to the attractiveness of the book among the great mass of readers'.[141] Regarding the book as a whole, he poignantly declares: 'We know of no romances half so interesting as the real "tales of terror" to be found scattered over these pages; and not a few of these, being American and Scotch, have never before made their appearance, in any shape at all, accessible to the general reader.'[142] While Dunlop's foray into forensic medicine was in essence a brief money-making venture before he left Edinburgh for the wilds of Upper Canada and the grandiose title of 'Warden of the Woods and Forests of the Canada Company', his work reveals how engagement with Blackwoodian literary forms and discourses could, in fact, be profitable to a medical man, particularly if his goal was popular appeal.[143]

'A Modern Pythagorean' and the Phrenological Imagination

Perhaps no medical man knew this so well as Robert Macnish. *The Anatomy of Drunkenness* (1827), *The Philosophy of Sleep* (1830), and *An Introduction to Phrenology* (1836) all went through multiple editions, and all were steeped in the type of medical subject matter that fascinated the *Blackwood's* coven: intoxication, the strange phenomena of sleep and dreaming, and phrenology. However, as 'champion of the Invisible World' in an age of 'utilitarian philosophy and materialism', *Blackwood's* walked a careful line between science and superstition – performing a balancing act of extremes.[144] An article of August 1818 decries John Ferriar's physiological explanation of apparitional experience in *An Essay Towards a Theory of Apparitions* (1813) for destroying

> the thrilling delight of a ghost-story by a Christmas fire-side, – the more exalted sense which a lurking tendency to superstitious apprehension adds to our relish of the sublime in poetry, – nay, the very pleasure which in some unaccountable manner mingles itself with the real terrors which situations such as above described are calculated to engender.[145]

However, an earlier article presents Ferriar's system in a more positive light. It offers a solution to the scepticism of the present generation in providing

> a new mode of judging evidence with respect to those supernatural matters, in which, without impeaching the truth of the narrator, or even the veracity of the eyes to whose evidence he appeals, you may ascribe his supposed facts to the effects of preconceived ideas acting upon faulty or diseased organs.[146]

It is this legitimising approach that is taken forward in a two-part series on 'A Few Passages Concerning Omens, Dreams, etc.' in 1840 and 1845, attributed to John Eagles (1783–1855), as well as in the 1847 series of 'Letters on the Truths Contained in Popular Superstitions' contributed by the London physician, physiologist and anatomist Herbert Mayo (1796–1852). Mayo attempts to explain a range of 'popular superstitions' through modern physiology and particularly mesmerism, and while endorsing, for example, a proto-spiritualist explanation of the phenomena of prophetic dreaming,[147] in the culminating article he is careful to declare that mesmerism 'contains absolutely nothing of the marvellous'.[148]

Like these Blackwoodian articles, Macnish's medico-popular writings enabled the post-Enlightenment reader to trespass into the murky realm of superstition and experience the thrill of the fantastic, while remaining (just) within the ever-expanding constraints of rationality. Knowing his audience well, in June 1829 Macnish sent an early manuscript of *The Philosophy of Sleep* to William Blackwood, asking if it is 'sufficiently popular in its character', and noting that Blackwood should find particularly interesting 'the sections on nightmare, on the phenomena of Dreaming and on the Prophetic power of Dreams'.[149] 'An Account of the Remarkable Case of Margaret Lyall' is recycled in a chapter on 'Protracted Sleep', and in the chapter 'On the Prophetic Power of Dreaming', Macnish cites a case first presented in *Blackwood's* in June 1826 as 'Remarkable Dream', addressed 'To the Editor of Blackwood's Magazine'.[150] Moir had suggested that Macnish 'give as many curious illustrations as possible, that being the way to make the book a popular one'.[151] Macnish might also have included extracts from the *Noctes* or from Hogg's 'The Shepherd's Calendar' series (1819–28), or perhaps from Maginn's 'The Man in the Bell' (1821), which includes a striking first-person description of dream-like hallucinations induced by extreme trauma, or Moir's own 'Singular Recovery from Death' (1821), which recounts a drunken dream vision. However, the Blackwoodian context did far more for Macnish than provide potential source material, and the tale of terror, in particular, served as an experimental template for the medical theorist and budding phrenologist.

The extreme situation that repeatedly prompts Macnish's many burlesques on the tale of terror is that of the philosophical observer who is frustrated by his own embodied subjectivity and thus his inability to read others. 'The Man with the Nose' of August 1826 is characteristic. The ludicrous horror of the tale is derived from the impenetrability of the significance of a nose. An unexpected guest startles a landlord and his guests with the great protuberance on his phiz: the party attempts to classify the nose, but 'it was neither an aquiline nose, nor a Roman nose, nor a snub nose . . . all philosophy was at fault'.[152] The landlord, eventually trapped alone with the man with the nose, falls into a nightmarish trance state, and the nose seems to grow to preposterous lengths – the impenetrability of its meaning exacerbating its horrific incongruity:

> It was this that tormented the looker-on. It was this that stood perpetually before his eyes, and would not be denied. The longer he looked at it the greater it grew, and the more his desire to look increased. Every moment it stretched out, and was at last a foot in length.[153]

As the mysterious man incessantly puffs upon his tobacco pipe, the landlord experiences visions similar to those described in *The Anatomy of Drunkenness*, in which, drawing upon a literary analogy, the intoxicating experience of tobacco is said to 'stand in the same relation to those of opium and wine . . . as Washington Irving to Lord Byron'. Macnish explains:

> If his fancy be unusually brilliant, or somewhat heated by previous drinking, he may see thousands of strange forms floating in the tobacco smoke. He may people it, according to his temperament, with agreeable or revolting images – with flowers and gems springing up, as in dreams, before him – or with reptiles, serpents, and the whole host of *diablerie*, skimming, like motes in the sunshine, amid its curling wreaths.[154]

The landlord in 'The Man with the Nose' is apparently of the latter temperament, as his imagery is diabolical rather than agreeable:

> [H]orrid forms were seen floating in the tobacco smoke – imps of darkness – snakes – crocodiles – toads – lizards, and all sorts of impure things. They leaped, and crawled, and flew with detestable hisses around – while the stranger grinned, and shook his head, and jabbered in an unearthly voice – his long nose, in the meantime, waving to and fro like a banner, while black demons, with tails and green eyes, sat astride upon it, screeching hideously. The spectacle was more than the landlord could endure, and he fell into a faint.[155]

The man with the nose does not manifest any diabolical behaviour within the tale, other than perhaps refusing to offer up any explanation of his unusual anatomy and sitting up rather late smoking and drinking. The visions are read as signs of the other man's character, but are in actuality indicative of the landlord's bodily and mental state.

This trope in Macnish's writing is undoubtedly related to his own unusually strong subjective colouring of the world. In January 1828 he writes to Moir regarding the visual imagery brought forth when he contemplates literary figures:

> Is it not singular that I can never think of Wilson without the idea of fresh mountain heath being presented to my mind; or of Barry Cornwall without thinking of a faded lily? When I think of you I have the image of a violet; and when of Hogg I cannot help seeing a huge boar, garlanded with roses, heather-bell, and wild thyme, rise up before me.[156]

While in this letter he exclaims that '[i]t is needless to reason on such psychological facts' as '[p]hilosophy will never explain them', a few years later he will interpret his experience in phrenological terms, as the result of a large organ of 'Comparison'.

In *An Introduction to Phrenology*, Macnish explains that the organ of Comparison 'enables us to trace resemblances and perceive analogies' and 'prompts to the use of figurative language'.[157] In a footnote to his delineation of individuals who exemplify a particularly large development of this organ, he notes:

> I know a gentleman in whom the activity of Comparison is so strong, that it prompts him to compare sounds with colours and names with physical objects. When a musical instrument is played, one tone seems to him to resemble blue, another green, another purple, and so on. The proper name, Combe, is associated in his mind with the figure of an urn, Simpson with an hour-glass, and Cox with a saw.[158]

In the second edition of *An Introduction of Phrenology* Macnish notes the relation of this gentleman's case in the 36th number of the *Phrenological Journal*. The gentleman is, in fact, Macnish himself.[159]

Today, Macnish's experience would be referred to as synaesthesia. Derived from the Greek for 'together perception', this phenomenon is neurologically defined by cross-modal interaction between senses within the cortical circuitry, and some evidence supports a structural differentiation of synaesthetes from the general population. An estimated 4.4 per cent of the population experience some form of synaesthesia as a normal part of daily perceptual experience, and only in recent decades has the existence of the condition received empirical support from the scientific community.[160] Macnish's organic justification of his condition is not entirely off-base according to modern scientific standards, but he expresses understandable confusion over his unusual subjective experience, which 'has existed since ever I recollect, and has puzzled myself as, I believe, it will do every other person'.[161] As is typical of phrenological evaluations, Macnish appeals to his writing style to evidence his particularly active faculty: 'In writing and reasoning, I feel at once that Comparison is the strongest faculty I have, and I believe there is no person who makes a greater use of similes and illustrations.'[162] Current research does indeed pose synaesthesia as evidence for a potential biological basis of figurative language, and speculations regarding an association between synaesthesia and a high level of creativity abound.[163] Macnish was not incorrect in his self-assessment. His success in producing medico-popular writing is largely derived from his ability to describe pathological experience through figurative language.

The tales of 'A Modern Pythagorean'– a mystical pseudonym derived from Macnish's first contribution to the magazine, 'The Metempsychosis', in May 1826 – often take their impetus from unreadable bodies that prompt vivid but indeterminate associative imagery.[164] In 'Who Can it Be?', a 'half a bottle of Port' and a dinner of 'oysters, devilled fowls, and macaroni' induces a trance-like state in which the narrator muses that a mysterious gentleman strolling through the courtyard of the University of Glasgow must, like himself, be a *'bon vivant'*, as '[s]uch cheeks, such a nose, such a double chin is not to be obtained for nothing. No, he understands living, well; he has read Apicius in the original, and is no doubt familiar with Meg Dods and Kitchiner. Perhaps he is Kitchiner himself.'[165] The conclusion of the tale of is one of painful irresolution. Similarly, in 'The Man with the Mouth', he is irresistibly distracted from reading 'Streams' – 'that exquisite creation of Christopher North's matchless pen' – by an unusual mouth possessed by a man in the Advocate's Library.[166] The stream of associations which the mysterious mouth prompts – that 'came upon [him] like a rainbow bursting out from the bosom of a

dark cloud – as a stream of sunshine at midnight – as the sound of the
Eolian harp in a summer eve' – echoes North's energetic associative
style and his insistence in 'Streams' upon the importance of physical
sensations – what 'the eye sees, and the ear hears' – in prompting
the imagination.[167] However, this aesthetic pleasure that 'touched the
heart, but not the head' is juxtaposed against the narrator's 'desire
to ascertain why such wonderful effects should spring from such a
cause'. He laments that 'being neither casuist nor phrenologist, I was
obliged to drop a subject, to which my powers were altogether une-
qual. I wondered, and was delighted; but what the remote springs of
such wonder and delight might be, baffled my philosophy, and set my
reasoning faculties at naught'.[168]

One of the key issues that finally attracted Macnish to phrenology
was the science's ability to create a strict correlation between external
appearances and the innate character of an individual. On one hand,
as George Combe (1788–1858), the leading populariser of phrenology in Scotland, indicates, 'Phrenology itself teaches its disciples that
we are variously constituted & hence cannot all see the same objects
in exactly the same light'[169] (a lesson Macnish really did not need
taught); on the other, the phrenologists continually insisted that their
methodology represented the first truly empirical science of the mind.
External reality – the bumps on the skull – corrected any imaginative
deviations from objective truth. In *An Introduction to Phrenology*
Macnish writes that his 'first ideas of Phrenology were obtained from
Dr. Gall himself', whose lectures he attended in Paris in 1825, but he
did not become a full convert to the science until 1833, when he sent
a cast of his own skull to the Edinburgh Phrenological Society for an
anonymous reading.[170] The experiment appears to have quelled all
doubt, but during the intervening period, he grappled with the valid-
ity of the doctrine.[171] These misgivings surface in prose tales that res-
olutely refuse to give way to the 'scientific' certitude of phrenology.
They at times critique the science – either for eliminating imaginative
potential or upon humanistic grounds – while also representing the
limitations of other methodologies, particularly linked to the Scottish philosophical tradition, including Hume and Smith's influential
theories of sympathetic exchange.

In the subtitle of *A Treatise of Human Nature* (1739–40), Hume
famously announces his 'attempt' 'to introduce the experimental
Method of Reasoning into moral subjects', or in other words, to

apply the inductive philosophic method of Newton and Bacon to the science of mind.[172] Hume's theory of sympathetic exchange is a crucial part of his attempt to study the mind of the other, which, unlike the material universe, is not accessible to public examination.[173] In the sympathetic exchange, the spectator views the signs of expressive feeling exhibited by the other, and from these impressions he forms ideas of the other's subjective experience.[174] These ideas are compared with the spectator's vivid idea of selfhood, resulting in the '[r]eembodiment of the idea of the other as an impression of our own'.[175] Smith's theory of sympathy in *The Theory of Moral Sentiments* (1759) revises the physiological immediacy of Hume's definition, and as Ian Duncan explains:

> But where Hume emphasises the involuntary, contagious force of sympathy activated by physical sensation, Smith invests sympathy with a disciplinary will gained on abstracting passion and reason from their chaotic origins in the body.[176]

Both formulations paradoxically stress the innate inability of man, with all his biases and preconceptions, to truly enter into the mind of the other, in other words, to become the idealised impartial spectator, whilst holding onto personal identity.[177] Stewart returns to the physiological immediacy of Hume's sympathetic engagement in his definition of sympathetic imitation.[178] Sympathetic imitation is the innate tendency in mankind to mimic the natural language – the expressions, gestures, and intonations of voice – of those around him and thus enter into phenomenological similitude. Stewart refers to the involuntary nature of sympathetic imitation, but carefully amends that he does not mean involuntary in a literal sense, but rather as a '*proneness*' capable of counteraction through 'the exercise of cool reflection, accompanied with a persevering and unremitting purpose directed to a particular end'.[179] As with Hume's definition, Stewart's sympathy elides individuality through its assimilatory powers.

The tale 'An Execution in Paris', published in *Blackwood's* in 1828, evidences Macnish's awareness of the complex inter-relations between the individual and society, the spectator and the other, and, in a more specialised fashion, the phrenological anatomist and the anatomical subject. As in Howison's 'Adventure in Havana', this tale inverts the case-history framing of the tale of terror, casting the narrator as medico-scientific observer. Based on his attendance at the execution of child-murderer Louis Auguste Papavoine in March 1825, while finishing his medical education in Paris, Macnish's description of grotesquely minute details would appeal to the Blackwoodian readership. However, the tale is driven forward by the narrator's reflections upon his attempt to philosophically observe the execution – to maintain a degree of distanced objectivity, which is constantly compromised by his scientifically dubious curiosity and the physiological intensity of his experience, which threatens to assimilate him into the emotive, voyeuristic, unphilosophical masses.

The narrator positions himself as a philosophical observer who is well aware of a certain voyeuristic barbarism accompanying the desire to witness a public execution, yet who nevertheless finds himself irresistibly drawn by an intense curiosity towards the uniquely French rendition of capital punishment:

> To my shame be it spoken, I wished to see an execution by the guillotine. There was a sort of sanguinary spell attached to this instrument, which irresistibly impelled me to witness one of its horrible triumphs.[180]

The term 'sanguinary' conjures up blood poured forth from the guillotine's victims and also underlines the physiological nature of the narrator's irresistible attraction to the machine:

> When I thought of it, the overwhelming tragedy of the Revolution was brought before my eyes – that Revolution which plunged Europe in seas of blood, and stamped an indelible impression upon the whole fabric of modern society.[181]

The intensity of the visual imagery associated with the idea of the guillotine – the phrase 'brought before my eyes' – indicates the conversion of idea into impression. This 'indelible impression' is felt not only within the individual body of the narrator, but also within the metaphorical body of society, for which the crowd of 'eighty thousand spectators' stands as representative. The open space immediately around the scaffold is a privileged place of spectatorship, reserved only for certain military men and their guests, and our philosophical observer is 'led into the area, and placed in front of the guillotine, not ten feet away from its dreadful presence'.[182]

The separation of the narrator's body from the heaving living body of the crowd sets up a dialectic of resistance: a movement towards 'the exercise of cool reflection' exposed by Stewart as the antidote to sympathetic assimilation.[183] Within this privileged place the narrator discovers that 'this machine is by no means so appalling to look at as the gallows'. The immediacy and relative humanity of the guillotine's actions, along with the knowledge that the 'noble and good have shed their blood in torrents beneath its edge', removes the element of disgrace associated with death by hanging. Without these associations of disgrace and the 'sickening imagery' of 'prolonged physical suffering', the fancy is free to speculate on the 'noble and enduring agony of the spirit, previous to the fatal hour'.[184] The disembodied death allows the spectator to participate in Smith's version of abstracted sympathetic exchange with the intended victim of the guillotine, and the narrator's description of Papavoine, who enters with an old Catholic priest, bespeaks this type of self-projective imaginative sympathy:

> Though pale and death-like, and seemingly impressed with the marks of sorrow and bad health, he exhibited no signs of terror or dismay. His demeanour was quiet and composed; and to the exhortations of his spiritual advisor he appeared to pay deep attention . . . had he died in a better cause, it would have been impossible not to admire his steady heroism.[185]

The calm delineation of the 'signs' of the prisoner's natural language is in stark contrast with the synchronised eruption of energy in the crowd:

> No sooner had the wretch entered the area appropriated for his fate, than a shout of deafening execration arose from the hitherto silent multitude. No preparatory murmurs of hatred and revenge preceded this ebullition of feeling. It sprung up simultaneously, and as if those from whom it proceeded were animated with one soul, and felt one pervading vengeance thrilling through their heart.[186]

However, at the critical point of the execution – the point at which Papavoine has 'committed himself to the hands of the executioner' – the crowd falls into a 'universal silence' of 'breathless awe', which 'was sickening to the last degree'. Reacting to the 'appalling' spectacle, the narrator's experience becomes intensely physical. His temporarily abstracted sympathy is re-embodied:

> While gazing upon the victim, my respiration was almost totally suspended – my heart beat violently, and a feeling of intense anxiety and suffocation pervaded my frame.[187]

His wilful withdrawal from the physiological immediacy of bodily reaction is overcome, and he is assimilated into the thronging masses. However, at the moment the condemned man's head is severed from the trunk, the narrator's stance as philosophical observer receives a new vitality. He is now able to look 'attentively to observe' the intimate details of the executed body – the self-projective sympathy that accompanied his examination of the natural signs of the living body dies as quickly as the severed corpse.[188] To his surprise, the trunk does not convulse at the instant of decapitation, but rather:

> lay from the first perfectly motionless, nor exhibited the slightest shudder – the least quivering – or the faintest indication that, the moment before, it was part of a sentient being, instinct with all the energies of life.[189]

The narrator lingers to view the transmutation of living flesh into scientific commodity: the head of Papavoine, after the blood is drained from it, is sent to the École de Médecine to be examined.

Once a degree of objectivity is achieved, a humanist critique develops. At the examination, the 'celebrated Doctor Gall' is present among the scientific men, as he 'was employed in investigating the developments of the head, and pointing them out to several of his pupils'.[190] The crucial distinction of phrenology from past philosophies of mind was the externalisation of mental faculties on the cranium, which made the human mind 'as open, accessible and easy to read, as the ages of the earth for a geologist working with volcanic rock'.[191] In essence, its methodology involved the collapsing of narrative and physical signs. The appendix to Macnish's *An Introduction to Phrenology* conflates an account of a convicted murderer's conduct just prior to execution with the post-mortem phrenological analysis of his skull:

The great size of Combativeness and Destructiveness (both 20) uncontrolled by his Benevolence, (which ranks only so high as 11,) and called into fierce action by liquor, easily accounts for the murder. . . . His great Love of Approbation, and his large Order, sufficiently explain the foppish freak of arranging his hair in curls at such a time, as well as the marked neatness of his dress as he appeared upon the scaffold.[192]

The minute details of this phrenological examination recorded in *An Introduction to Phrenology* are in stark contrast to the single sentence devoted to Gall's phrenological evaluation of Papavoine in 'An Execution in Paris'. While it is possible that Macnish simply no longer recalls the minute details of the evaluation, or perhaps did not pay close attention at the time, this evasion may also be read as a negative commentary on phrenology (as well as perhaps on French pathological anatomy more generally). With the shocking rapidity of decapitation, the transition from a sentient being, capable of eliciting sympathy and wrath, to an insentient object, the description of which evinces no significant indications of an internal life, is instantaneous. This eludes the phrenologist: Gall examines the severed head, drained of all its blood, in the same way he might examine a living cranium.

Despite such a close convergence between his scientific interests and his literary experiments, by the end of his life Macnish came to view the latter as inherently of lesser value than the former. In his last letter to Moir, before his untimely death on the 16th of January 1837, Macnish distinguishes the second edition of *An Introduction to Phrenology* as 'the best of my works'.[193] A reviewer of the book for the *Phrenological Journal* explains that Macnish had studied

with intense interest Mr [George] Combe's work on the Constitution of Man, and informed the writer of the present notice, that the book had opened up to his mind a new view of life and the world, and given to his thoughts and aspirations higher interests and aims than they had ever before possessed. His pursuits in the region of fancy then appeared to him unprofitable, he felt the superiority of the principles of science, and stated that he was conscious of a revolution taking place in his whole mental condition.[194]

This supposed final denigration of Macnish's 'pursuits in the region of fancy' (if we read it as reliable) may be linked, in part, to the negative reception of *The Philosophy of Sleep*, and more broadly, to the growing sense of incommensurability between literary and medico-scientific cultures at this time.

According to Macnish's letters to Moir and Blackwood, the work sold well in the first months, with half of the original print run of 2,000 selling in the first five months.[195] However, the medical community saw little scientific value in it. A reviewer for *The Lancet* complains that, although Macnish denies the prophetic power of dreaming, 'he has related some very singular cases (of one of which he was himself the subject) which would almost induce a belief that such was the case'.[196] Both *The Lancet* and the *London Medical Gazette* viewed the book's title as misleading, its observations and theories as unoriginal and even plagiaristic, and its composition as over-hasty. Such praise as was offered was mixed. While noting some potential usefulness to the general reader, *The Lancet* labelled it 'rather an amusing than an instructive production' and characterised its observations as 'poetical' rather than 'philosophical'.[197] Similarly, the reviewer for the *London Medical Gazette* writes:

> His attempts to combine physic, philosophy, and entertainment, have been in general successful; but it is to be confessed, at the same time, that both his physic and his philosophy have always been of that airy and popular kind which presents the most attractive front to the numerous and respectable class of light readers.[198]

The reception from the lay community was comparable. While Bell's *Edinburgh Literary Journal* praises Macnish's investigation as both rousing to 'the imagination of the poet' and appealing 'to the judgment of the philosopher', it does 'not regard this work as likely to raise his fame in the estimation of men of science'.[199]

When a second edition was called for in the spring of 1833, Macnish was eager for the opportunity to make improvements. He writes to Moir in April 1833: 'As the Book stands I am somewhat ashamed [of] it, and must do my best to make it do its author more credit.'[200] While his descriptions of the various phenomenologies of altered states of consciousness maintain their poetical character, the literary mottos that had prefaced each chapter are removed, since they are 'out of place in a scientific work'.[201] In a new chapter devoted to

'Spectral Illusions', Macnish discounts second sight and fairy encounters, attributes them to 'ignorance', 'superstition', and an 'excited brain', and enhances the scientific character of the text with the addition of more case histories and phrenological explanations.[202] Thus, 'The Modern Pythagorean' – one of the greatest lovers of Blackwoodian mysticism – devoted his final years to unfolding the mysteries of the human mind through the science of phrenology.

Blackwoodian Medicine

Medical contributors to *Blackwood's* found themselves in a curious position. Many of the medico-scientific developments that fascinated Blackwoodian writers – pathological anatomy, phrenology and forensic medicine – were central to efforts to make both the science of the mind and medicine more objective and authoritative. However, part of Maga's appeal was its celebration of that which lies just beyond 'the empire of science',[203] and this is paralleled by its own overarching insistent illusiveness – its 'parodies, ventriloquism, reversals of "ordinary" signification, confessions of "Balaam", mystifications of signature, hoaxing, and deceptively referential discourse'.[204] Jon Klancher has argued that *Blackwood's* writers continually rhetorically gesture towards an '"inaccessible nucleus" of meaning' that is 'beyond the grasp of verbal signs', presenting readers with an 'ever-receding Mind just beyond its grasp'.[205] Such hermeneutic illusiveness presents potential difficulties for a profession devoted to ever-increasing legibility of the signs of the body and the mind. However, one key driver of *Blackwood's* medico-popular writing was the reclamation of phenomena beyond the grasp of the anatomy table or the statisticians' tabulations. As De Quincey indicates in his 'Suspiria de Profundis' in *Blackwood's* in 1845: 'The true object in my "Opium Confessions" is not the naked physiological theme . . . but those wandering musical variations upon the theme – those parasitical thoughts, feelings, and digressions, which climb up with bells and blossoms round about the arid stock.'[206]

Klancher also discusses a negative hermeneutic active in *Blackwood's*, in which 'the social mind forms and collapses distinctions, the power of its critical act becoming the measure of its own distinction from all the social signs it encounters'.[207] The medical profession – defined by its powers of interpreting the otherness of disease and deviance – contributed to this hermeneutic. Forensic medicine and phrenology were sign-reading methodologies capable of diagnosing deviance and perhaps even of understanding national character. In his review of *The Anatomy of Drunkenness* Wilson celebrates Macnish's text as 'a moral dissertation on the nature, causes, and effects of one of the most deplorable and pernicious vices than can degrade and afflict all the ongoings of social life' and declares: 'Drunkard, stand forward, that we may have a look at you, and draw your picture.'[208] The picture inverts Wilson's proto-Kailyard ideal of pastoral Scottish identity: a 'scholar of bright parts' falls prey to drunkenness, ministers and medical men disgrace their families and are 'found drowned in pits or pools – or smothered in barley-mows – or suffocated in ditches – or found suspended in their "braces" on trees', and the worst case of all that 'well-educated, moral, religious Scotland, can show, in the bosom of her bonny banks and braes', turns out to be a drunken 'Elder of the Kirk'.[209]

Despite the synergies this chapter has explored, the latter part of Macnish's career exemplifies the growing sense of incommensurability between literary and medico-scientific cultures at this time. As the next chapter will detail, both he and Moir were anxious to keep their identities as authors of imaginative literature and as surgeons separate. However, if *Blackwood's* enabled the development of a form of medico-popular fiction that countered what was perceived as the reductive, unfeeling, unimaginative tendencies of medico-scientific and philosophic thinking and writing, the magazine also constructed a new ideal of the physician or surgeon as man-of-letters and humanitarian, who reunites intellect and feeling through his engagement with literary culture.

Notes

1. [Mr. Vary], 'Essays on Cranioscopy, Craniology, Phrenology, &c. By Sir Toby Tickletoby, Bart.', *BEM*, 10 (August 1821, Part II), 73–82 (p. 73).
2. Ibid. p. 76.
3. Ibid. p. 80.

4. 'Introductory Statement', *PJ*, 1 (1823), iii–xxxi (pp. xvii–xviii).
5. [W. E. Aytoun], 'Mesmeric Mountebanks', *BEM*, 60 (August 1846), 223–37 (p. 223).
6. Connell, *Romanticism, Economics, and the Question of 'Culture'*, p. 11.
7. Pomata, 'The Medical Case Narrative: Distant Reading of an Epistemic Genre', p. 2.
8. Robert Macnish to D. M. Moir, 13 August 1827, NLS Watson Collection, MS 583 (828), fols 234–35.
9. Moir, *The Modern Pythagorean*, vol. 1, pp. 51–2.
10. Moir appears to be referencing the same 'reading public at large' that Coleridge famously declared benefited from the 'epoch in periodical criticism' initiated by the *Edinburgh Review* (Coleridge, *Biographia Literaria*, vol. 2, p. 108).
11. Moir, *The Modern Pythagorean*, vol. 1, p. 36, p. 37.
12. For examples of the positive reception of the first edition, see 'The Philosophy of Drunkenness', *MM*, 3.18 (June 1827), 601–14; 'Macnish's *The Anatomy of Drunkenness*', *Literary Chronicle*, 415 (April 1827), 262–4; 'Macnish's *The Anatomy of Drunkenness*', *The Lancet*, 8 (5 May 1827), 149–55.
13. Macnish, *The Anatomy of Drunkenness* (1827), p. 1.
14. Trotter, *An Essay, Medical, Philosophical, and Chemical on Drunkenness*, p. 26.
15. Ibid. p. 14.
16. Macnish, *The Anatomy of Drunkenness* (1827), p. 6.
17. [John Wilson], 'Anatomy of Drunkenness', *BEM*, 23 (April 1828), 481–99 (p. 489).
18. Robert Macnish to D. M. Moir, 2 October 1827, NLS, Acc. 9856, No. 49; Vickers, *Coleridge and the Doctors 1795–1806*, p. 41.
19. Richardson, *British Romanticism and the Science of the Mind*, pp. 51–2.
20. Macnish, *The Anatomy of Drunkenness*, 2nd edn (1828), pp. 79–82.
21. Robert Macnish to D. M. Moir, 5 January 1828, NLS Acc. 9856, No. 49.
22. De Quincey, *Confessions*, in *The Works of Thomas De Quincey*, vol. 2, p. 9, p. 10, p. 11.
23. Leask, *British Romantic Writers and the East*, pp. 172–3.
24. Macnish, *The Anatomy of Drunkenness* (1827), pp. 22–3.
25. Higgins, 'Imaging the Exotic: De Quincey and Lamb in the *London Magazine*', p. 290.
26. De Quincey, *Confessions*, in *The Works of Thomas De Quincey*, vol. 2, p. 13.

27. Symonds, *De Quincey to His Publishers*, pp. 57–8, as cited in Lindrop, 'Textual History', in *The Works of Thomas De Quincey*, vol. 2, p. 3.
28. Ibid. p. 3. See also Higgins, 'Imaging the Exotic: De Quincey and Lamb in the *London Magazine*', p. 290; Morrison, 'Opium-Eaters and Magazine Wars'.
29. De Quincey, *Confessions*, in *The Works of Thomas De Quincey*, vol. 2, p. 13. See Robert Morrison's discussion of the continuing relations between Wilson and De Quincey after the latter decamped to the *London Magazine*, in Morrison's co-edited volume *Romanticism and Blackwood's Magazine*.
30. [William Howison?], 'Essays on the Lake School of Poetry. No. II', *BEM*, 4 (December 1818), 257–63 (p. 257).
31. [Lockhart], *Peter's Letters*, vol. 1, p. 178.
32. Ibid. p. 177, p. 178, p. 179.
33. Levin, *The Romantic Art of Confession*, p. 26.
34. Ibid. pp. 29–30.
35. [Lockhart], *Peter's Letters*, vol. 1, p. 176, p. 177.
36. On the inclusion of 'remarkable' cases in the *Gentleman's Magazine*, see Porter, 'Lay Medical Knowledge in the Eighteenth Century', pp. 142–3. Medical cases were also frequently detailed within the monthly medical reports of the *Monthly Magazine*, particularly as the reports progressively shifted from an empirical tabulation of disease statistics to discussion of the individual reporters' encounters with disease in that particular month.
37. See, for example, 'Curious Account of the hanging and recovery of Margaret Dickson', *SM*, 70 (December 1808), 905–6; 'Particulars of the Case of Ann Moore, called the Fasting-Woman of Tutbury. By A. Henderson, M.D. Physician to the Westminster General Dispensary', *SM*, 74 (January 1813), 32–8; 'Extraordinary Instance of SELF CRUCIFIXION. From the Pamphleteer. No. 6', *SM*, 76 (August 1814), 602–06; and 'Remarkable Cases of the Reunion of Members separated from the Human Body. By William Balfour, M.D. (From the Edinburgh Medical Journal)', *SM*, 76 (December 1814), 887–92.
38. For a critical overview of Molyneux's philosophical case, see Kennedy, *Revising the Clinic*, pp. 30–53.
39. For extracts from the Stewart/Jeffrey debate, see Flynn, *Enlightenment Scotland*, pp. 76–88.
40. Morrison and Baldick, 'Introduction', pp. xiv–xv.
41. Ibid. p. xv; see also Worthington, *The Rise of the Detective*, pp. 6–45.
42. Killick, *British Short Fiction in the Early Nineteenth Century*, p. 25.
43. Sucksmith, 'The Secret of Immediacy', p. 146.

44. Morrison and Baldick, 'Introduction', p. xv.

45. Killick, '*Blackwood's* and the Boundaries of the Short Story', in Morrison and Roberts (eds), *Romanticism and Blackwood's Magazine*, p. 170.

46. Further examples of this third-person narrative mode may be found in an early series of articles on animal magnetism: [Robert Gordon], 'Observations on Animal Magnetism', *EMM*, 1 (September 1817), 563–7; [Robert Gordon], 'On the Present State of Animal Magnetism in Germany', *BEM*, 2 (October 1817), 36–8; [Robert Gordon], 'The German Somnambulists and Miss M'Avoy', *BEM*, 2 (January 1818), 437–43.

47. James Brewster, 'Remarkable Case of Margaret Lyall, Who Continued in a State of Sleep Nearly Six Weeks', *EMM*, 1 (April 1817), 61–4 (p. 64).

48. Ibid. p. 64.

49. Ibid. p. 63.

50. [John Wilson], 'Remarkable Preservation from Death at Sea', *BEM*, 2 (February 1818), 490–4 (p. 490).

51. Ibid. p. 490.

52. Ibid. p. 493.

53. 'Colter's Escape from the Blackfeet Indians', *BEM*, 3 (April 1818), 45–6 (p. 45).

54. [John Wilson], 'Extracts from Gosschen's Diary', *BEM*, 3 (August 1818), 596–8 (p. 598).

55. [J. G. Lockhart], 'Christian Wolf, A True Story. – From the German', *BEM*, 3 (September 1818), 679–89 (p. 679).

56. On this trend for case histories in the *Edinburgh Medical and Surgical Journal* specifically, see Atkinson, 'The Evolution of Medical Research Writing from 1735 to 1985'.

57. [Lockhart], 'Christian Wolf', p. 680.

58. Foucault, *Birth of the Clinic*, pp. 176–7.

59. [Lockhart], 'Christian Wolf', p. 679.

60. Ibid. p. 680.

61. De Quincey, *Confessions*, in *The Works of Thomas De Quincey*, vol. 2, p. 87.

62. [John Galt], 'The Buried Alive', *BEM*, 10 (October 1821), 262–4 (p. 263, p. 262).

63. Ibid. p. 263. I borrow this phase from Schoenfield's title, 'The Taste for Violence in *Blackwood's Magazine*', in Morrison and Roberts (eds), *Romanticism and Blackwood's Magazine*, pp. 187–202.

64. De Quincey, 'On Murder Considered as One of the Fine Arts', in *The Works of Thomas De Quincey*, vol. 6, p. 126.

65. 'On the Pleasures of "Body-Snatching"', *MM*, 3 (April 1827), 355–65 (p. 355, p. 359, p. 364).

66. [Sir Edward Bruce Hamley], 'A Recent Confession of an Opium Eater', *BEM*, 80 (December 1856), 629–36 (p. 635).

67. Kennedy, *Revising the Clinic*, pp. 54–5.

68. [Walter Scott or William Laidlaw], 'Narrative of a Fatal Event', *BEM*, 2 (March 1818), 630–5 (p. 632).

69. Ibid. p. 633.

70. De Quincey, 'Appendix', in *The Works of Thomas De Quincey*, vol. 2, p. 81, pp. 81–2.

71. Logan, *Nerves and Narratives*, p. 73.

72. For a full account of this genre, see Hawkins, *Reconstructing Illness*.

73. Milligan, 'Morphine-Addicted Doctors, the English Opium-Eater, and Embattled Medical Authority', p. 543.

74. 'Medical Article. No. I', *LM*, 1 (January 1820), 95–6; 'Medical Article. No. II', *LM*, 1 (February 1820), 179–80; 'Medical Article. No. III. On Temperature as Affecting Health', *LM*, 1 (March 1820), 314–16; 'Medical Article. No. IV. On Clothing', *LM*, 1 (April 1820), 451–4.

75. [Samuel Warren], 'Passages from the Diary of a Late Physician. Chap. VII. The Spectre-Smitten', *BEM*, 29 (February 1831), 361–75 (p. 361).

76. Morrison, 'John Howison of "Blackwood's Magazine"', p. 191; Jarrells, 'Tales of the Colonies: *Blackwood's*, Provincialism, and British Interests Abroad', in Morrison and Roberts (eds), *Romanticism and Blackwood's Magazine*, p. 274.

77. McMullen, '"A Wrong Port": Colonial Havana under Northern Eyes', p. 68.

78. [John Howison], 'Adventure in Havana', *BEM*, 9 (June 1821), 305–12 (p. 309).

79. McMullen, '"A Wrong Port": Colonial Havana under Northern Eyes', p. 75.

80. [Howison], 'Adventure in Havana', p. 305, p. 306. As Alan Bewell notes, the image of the corpse floating back out of the water is common in colonial military disease narratives and is indicative of the human cost of empire (*Romanticism and Colonial Disease*, pp. 66–130). Ian Duncan has read the recurrent trope of the 'upright corpse', the soulless body rising from the grave or deathbed, in Hogg's corpus as a metaphor for the false revival of Scottish culture as led by Scott (*Scott's Shadow*, pp. 183–214), but in the wider Blackwoodian context, the image is one of guilt and transgression, broadly and variously conceived.

81. D. M. Moir to William Blackwood, dated 20 June 1820 [corrected as 1821], NLS MS 4007, fols 177–8.

82. [Howison], 'Adventure in Havana', p. 306.

83. For a full overview, see Tröhler, *"To Improve the Evidence of Medicine"*.

84. Ibid. p. 21. In relation to this gradual trend in the *Edinburgh Medical and Surgical Journal* specifically, see Atkinson, 'The Evolution of Medical Research Writing from 1735 to 1985'.

85. John Howison, 'On the Remote Causes of Death', *Records of the Royal Medical Society*, 75 (1816–17), fols 133–42 (fol. 134).

86. Ibid. fol. 137.

87. [Howison], 'Adventure in Havana', p. 306.

88. Howison, 'On the Remote Causes of Death', fol. 135.

89. Ibid. fol. 136. For fictive examples, see 'Sablegrove', in *Tales of the Colonies*, vol. 1, pp. 221–342, vol. 2, pp. 3–79, and 'The Cantonment of Seroor' in *Foreign Scenes and Travelling Recreations*, vol. 2, p. 168.

90. Howison, 'Foreign Adventure', in *Foreign Scenes and Travelling Recreations*, vol. 2, p. 118, p. 137.

91. For an enthusiastic review, see [John Galt], 'Howison's Canada', *BEM*, 10 (December 1821), 537–45. The *Edinburgh Review* likewise praised the work, but noted that Howison is not a 'scientific traveller' ([Hugh Murray], 'Howison's Upper Canada', *ER*, 37 (June 1822), 249–68 (p. 255)).

92. Emerson, *Essays on David Hume, Medical Men and the Scottish Enlightenment*, pp. 188–93.

93. Johann Peter Frank, 'Description of Edinburgh: with an Account of the present State of its Medical School. From the German of Frank', *SM*, 71 (February 1809), 94–8 (p. 95).

94. Hart, *Lockhart as Romantic Biographer*, p. 54; Leask, *Curiosity and the Aesthetics of Travel Writing*, p. 5.

95. Hart, *Lockhart as Romantic Biographer*, p. 54.

96. [John Howison], 'Vanderbrummer; or, the Spinosist', *BEM*, 10 (December 1821), 501–8 (p. 501).

97. Ibid. p. 501.

98. Tröhler, *"To Improve the Evidence of Medicine"*, p. 21.

99. McCullough, *John Gregory's Writings on Medical Ethics and Philosophy of Medicine*, p. 130. On philosophical medicine in Germany, see Risse's essays: 'Kant, Schelling, and the Early Search for a Philosophical "Science" of Medicine in Germany'; '"Philosophical" Medicine in Nineteenth-Century Germany'.

100. John Thomson, 'Has Theory tended to promote or retard the Science of MEDICINE?', *Records of the Royal Medical Society, commencing in March 1808*, 61 (1808–9), fols 41–60 (fol. 59).

101. 'Inquiries concerning the Intellectual Powers, and the investigation of Truth. By John Abercrombie, M.D.', *EMSJ*, 35 (January 1831), 401–25 (p. 405).
102. Hampshire, *Spinoza and Spinozism*, p. 32.
103. Damasio, *Looking for Spinoza*.
104. [Howison], 'Vanderbrummer; or, the Spinosist', p. 502.
105. Ibid. p. 503.
106. Ibid. p. 504.
107. Ibid. p. 505.
108. Ibid. p. 505, p. 507.
109. Ibid. p. 506.
110. Ibid. p. 508.
111. Thomas Beddoes, *A Letter to the Right Honourable Sir Joseph Banks . . . on the Causes and Removal of the Prevailing Discontents, Imperfections, and Abuses, in Medicine* (London: Richard Phillips, 1808), p. 55, p. 72, as cited in Porter, 'Plutus or Hygeia?; Thomas Beddoes and the Crisis of Medical Ethics in Britain at the Turn of the Nineteenth Century', in Baker, Porter, and Porter (eds), *The Codification of Medical Morality*, p. 83, p. 84; [Maginn], 'Letter to Pierce Egan, Esq.', p. 671.
112. [Lockhart], *Peter's Letters to his Kinsfolk*, vol. 2, p. 150, p. 151.
113. Ibid. vol. 3, p. 139.
114. Walter Scott to Joanna Baillie, 10 February 1822, in H. J. C. Grierson et al. (eds), *The Letters of Sir Walter Scott*, centenary edn, 12 vols (London: Constable & Co., 1932–37), vol. 7, p. 59.
115. William Howison, 'An Essay on the Arrangement of the Categories. By William Howison', *BEM*, 11 (March 1822), 308–16 (p. 308, p. 309).
116. William Howison, *The Contest of the Twelve Nations*, p. 11, p. 13.
117. 'The Contest of the Twelve Nations, &c.', *PJ*, 3 (1825–6), 628–34 (p. 634).
118. *Edinburgh Advertiser*, 14 November 1823, as quoted in Graham, *The Tiger of Canada West*, p. 36.
119. 'Prospectus of a Course of Lectures on Forensic Medicine', p. 4; Graham, *The Tiger of Canada West*, p. 36.
120. Graham, *The Tiger of Canada West*, p. 18.
121. Ibid. p. 34; [William Dunlop], 'Calcutta. Chap. VIII. The Supreme Court', *BEM*, 13 (April 1823), 443–9 (p. 448).
122. Crawford, 'A scientific profession', p. 204.
123. Ibid. p. 208. See also Watson, *Forensic Medicine in Western Society*, pp. 46–71.

124. Crowther and White, *On soul and conscience*, pp. 5–26; White, 'Training medical policemen'.
125. Robert Gooch to John Murray, no date, NLS MS 40458.
126. [John Hope], 'Hints for Jurymen', *BEM*, 13 (June 1823), 673–85 (p. 674).
127. Worthington, *The Rise of the Detective*, pp. 30–45.
128. Ibid. p. 30, p. 40.
129. William Dunlop, 'Introductory Lecture', in *Lectures on Medical Jurisprudence* [1823–4], 2 vols, Harvard Medical Library in the Francis A. Countway Library of Medicine, Rare Books H MS b37, vol. 1 [unpaginated folios].
130. Ibid.
131. [J. G. Lockhart], 'Beck and Dunlop on Medical Jurisprudence', *BEM*, 17 (March 1825), 351–2 (p. 351).
132. [William Maginn], 'Canada. By Tiger – Galt – Picken', *FM*, 5 (July 1832), 635–42 (p. 636).
133. Elizabeth Baigent, 'Dunlop, William (1792–1848)', *ODNB*, available at http://www.oxforddnb.com/view/article/37377?docPos=3 (last accessed 16 June 2016).
134. Dunlop, *Lectures on Medical Jurisprudence*, vol. 1.
135. Ibid. vol. 2.
136. Ibid.
137. Ibid.
138. Ibid.
139. Schoenfield, 'The Taste for Violence in *Blackwood's Magazine*'.
140. William Dunlop to William Blackwood, 11 September 1824, NLS MS 4012, fols 111–12.
141. [Lockhart], 'Beck and Dunlop on Medical Jurisprudence', p. 352, p. 351.
142. Ibid. p. 352.
143. Graham, *The Tiger of Canada West*, p. 45.
144. [Aytoun], 'Mesmeric Mountebanks', p. 223.
145. [John Herman Merivale], 'Phantasmagoriana; Tales of the Dead, Principally Translated from the French', *BEM*, 3 (August 1818), 589–96 (p. 590).
146. [William Laidlaw], 'Phantasmagoria', *BEM*, 3 (May 1818), 211–15 (pp. 211–12).
147. [Herbert Mayo], 'Letters on the Truths Contained in Popular Superstitions. No. IV.– Reals Ghosts, and Second-Sight, V.– Trance and Sleepwalking', *BEM*, 61 (May 1847), 541–55 (p. 541).
148. [Herbert Mayo], 'Letters on the Truths Contained in Popular Superstitions. No. VII.– Objects to be Gained through the Artificial Induction of Trance, *BEM*, 62 (August 1847), 166–77 (p. 169).

149. Robert Macnish to William Blackwood, 3 June 1829, NLS MS 4025, fols 124–5. Blackwood did not publish the text, and, interestingly, Macnish later claims he 'disliked' it (Robert Macnish to D. M. Moir, 22 October 1831, NLS Acc. 9856, No. 49).

150. Macnish, *The Philosophy of Sleep* (1830), pp. 215–17, pp. 109–11. The second edition of Macnish's text includes a second case extracted from *Blackwood's*, as well as a case from *Fraser's* (Macnish, *The Philosophy of Sleep*, 2nd edn (1834), pp. 104–5, pp. 182–3).

151. Moir, *The Modern Pythagorean*, vol. 1, p. 136.

152. [Robert Macnish], 'The Man with the Nose', *BEM*, 20 (August 1826), 159–63 (pp. 159–60).

153. Ibid. p. 162.

154. Macnish, *The Anatomy of Drunkenness*, 2nd edn (1828), p. 75.

155. [Macnish], 'The Man with the Nose', pp. 162–3.

156. Robert Macnish to D. M. Moir, 5 January 1828, NLS Acc. 9856, No. 49.

157. Macnish, *An Introduction to Phrenology*, p. 115.

158. Ibid. p. 116.

159. See Moir, *The Modern Pythagorean*, vol. 1, p. 270, pp. 272–306.

160. Hochel and Milán, 'Synaesthesia: The Existing State of Affairs'.

161. [Robert Macnish, James Simpson, and Robert Cox], 'Natural Dispositions and Talents Inferred from a Cast of a Head; with Subsequent Correspondence Relative to Some Peculiarities', *PJ*, 8 (1832–4), 206–23 (p. 216).

162. Ibid. p. 216.

163. Hochel and Milán, 'Synaesthesia: The Existing State of Affairs', p. 113, p. 100.

164. For a reading of 'The Metempsychosis', see Coyer, 'Phrenological Controversy and the Medical Imagination: "A Modern Pythagorean" in *Blackwood's Edinburgh Magazine*', in Coyer and Shuttleton (eds), *Scottish Medicine and Literary Culture, 1726–1832*, pp. 184–9.

165. [Robert Macnish], 'Who Can It Be?', *BEM*, 22 (October 1827), 432–7 (p. 432).

166. [Robert Macnish], 'The Man with the Mouth', *BEM*, 23 (May 1828), 597–601 (p. 597).

167. Ibid. p. 597; [John Wilson], 'Streams', *BEM*, 9 (April 1826), 375–403 (p. 390).

168. [Macnish], 'The Man with the Mouth', p. 597.

169. George Combe to Samuel Hibbert, 18 March 1824, NLS MS 7383, fol. 24.

170. Macnish, *An Introduction to Phrenology*, p. v.

171. 'Biographical Sketch of Robert Macnish, esq., LL.D.', p. 22.

172. For a facsimile of the original title page, see Hume, *A Treatise of Human Nature*, p. 33.
173. Ibid. pp. 45–6.
174. In Hume's theory, impressions and ideas differ only in 'the degrees of force and liveliness, with which they strike upon the mind, and make their way into our thought or consciousness' (ibid. p. 49).
175. Duncan, *Scott's Shadow*, p. 268.
176. Duncan, 'Hume and the Scottish Enlightenment', p. 76.
177. For further, see Daffron, *Romantic Doubles* and Duncan, *Scott's Shadow*, pp. 264–72.
178. Duncan, *Scott's Shadow*, p. 270; Stewart, *Elements of the Philosophy of the Human Mind*, vol. 3, pp. 153–244.
179. Ibid. p. 170.
180. [Robert Macnish], 'An Execution in Paris', *BEM*, 24 (December 1828), 785–8 (p. 785).
181. Ibid. p. 785.
182. Ibid. p. 786.
183. Stewart, *Elements of the Philosophy of the Human Mind*, vol. 3, p. 170.
184. Ibid. p. 786.
185. Ibid. p. 787.
186. Ibid. p. 787.
187. Ibid. p. 787.
188. Ibid. p. 788.
189. Ibid. p. 788.
190. Ibid. p. 788.
191. Stack, *Queen Victoria's Skull*, p. 46.
192. Macnish, *An Introduction to Phrenology*, p. 171.
193. Robert Macnish to D. M. Moir, 6 December 1836, NLS Acc. 9856, No. 50.
194. 'Macnish's *An Introduction to Phrenology*', *PJ*, 10 (1836–7), 552–6 (p. 553).
195. Robert Macnish to William Blackwood, 27 February 1831, NLS MS 4030, fols 131–2.
196. 'Macnish's *The Philosophy of Sleep*', *The Lancet*, 15 (19 February 1831), 673–9 (p. 675).
197. Ibid. p. 673.
198. 'Dr. Macnish on *The Philosophy of Sleep*', *LMG*, 7 (20 November 1830), 246–9 (p. 247).
199. 'Macnish's *The Philosophy of Sleep*', *Edinburgh Literary Journal*, 2 (16 October 1830), 238–9.
200. Robert Macnish to D. M. Moir, 9 April 1833, NLS Acc. 9856, No. 50.

201. Robert Macnish to D. M. Moir, 3 February 1834, NLS Acc. 9856, No. 50.
202. Macnish, *The Philosophy of Sleep*, 2nd edn (1834), pp. 241–75 (p. 259, p. 260).
203. On the derivation of the familiar name Maga, see David Finkelstein, 'Selling Blackwood's Magazine, 1817–1834', in Morrison and Roberts (eds), *Romanticism and Blackwood's Magazine*, pp. 69–86 (p. 70).
204. [Lockhart], *Peter's Letters*, vol. 1, p, 177; Parker, *Literary Magazines and British Romanticism*, p. 136.
205. Klancher, *The Making of English Reading Audiences*, p. 59, p. 58, p. 61.
206. De Quincey, 'Suspiria de Profundis: Being a Sequel to the Confessions of an English Opium-Eater', in *The Works of Thomas De Quincey*, vol. 15, p. 135.
207. Klancher, *The Making of English Reading Audiences*, p. 74.
208. [John Wilson], 'Anatomy of Drunkenness', *BEM*, 23 (April 1828), 481–99 (p. 481, p. 494).
209. Ibid. p. 495, p. 496.

Chapter 3

'Delta': The Construction of a Nineteenth-Century Literary Surgeon

Delta. . . . Your judgment, and that of other enlightened men, have [sic] confirmed my own, that such occasional relaxation, as the study of elegant literature affords, from the not unsevere and rarely intermitting labours of a profession, of which I conscientiously endeavour to discharge the duties, to the best of my skill and knowledge, so far from either incapacitating or disinclining my mind for such labours and such duties, does greatly strengthen both its moral and intellectual energies.

. . .

North. Heavens! can any studies be idle in a physician – in a medical man – that inevitably lead to elevation of spirit, breathing into it tenderness and humanity? Will he be a less thoughtful visitant at the sick or dying bed, who from such studies has gathered knowledge of all the beatings of the human heart, and all the workings of the human imagination, at such times so wild and so bewildering, aye, often even beyond the range of poetry, in those delirious dreams?[1]

In August 1830 David Macbeth Moir, pen-named 'Delta', made his singular debut as a character in the *Noctes Ambrosianæ*. 'The Modern Pythagorean', aka Robert Macnish, also features for the first and only time in the series. In a letter to Blackwood in July 1830, Macnish notes that 'When I saw Professor Wilson in Edinburgh he spoke of introducing a new character into the Noctes viz. The Modern Pythagorean', but laments:

Had I been a free agent in this matter I should have felt proud beyond measure in being placed there, but the people in this place are such an infernal set of apes that they look with an evil eye upon a medical man who has any thing to do with literature unless it be upon professional subjects.[2]

In the same letter Macnish tentatively grants Blackwood permission to print the 'Noctes', if it has already been written, 'for it would be out of the question that on my account the article should be spoilt', but expresses his desire that 'something could be said in the Noctes about the execrable absurdity of that doctrine, which supposes that a person cannot excel both in literature and professional subjects: the very idea is a disgrace to the intellect of the age'.[3] North's enthusiastic endorsement of Moir's extra-professional endeavours answers Macnish's request. However, it also responds to wider cultural needs at this particular point in Scottish medical and literary history. The reputation of the medical profession was at a low ebb in Edinburgh when this 'Noctes' was written, and the need for 'tenderness and humanity' particularly evident. The West Port murders had come to light in 1828, and Moir's portrayal as a literary surgeon is directly linked to this macabre chapter in Edinburgh's medical history.

The anatomy murders of William Burke and William Hare were a favoured topic in the 'Noctes', and North made it 'no secret' that he believed Dr Robert Knox was guilty of complicity.[4] Perhaps the most trenchant critique may be found in the 'Noctes' of March 1829, in which North decries the cheers that met Knox from his students when he returned to the dissecting rooms, as 'calculated – whatever their effect on more thinking minds – to confirm in those of the populace the conviction that they are all a gang of murderers together, and determined to insult, in horrid exultation, all the deepest feelings of humanity'.[5] Moir also worried about the damage done to the reputation of the medical profession by Knox and his supporters. In January 1829 he writes to Macnish:

> [N]othing ever gave me viler opinion of medical morality, than the conduct of the Profession on this atrociously memorable occasion; and nothing, I am sure, since the days that old Herophilus dissected living men, has ever occurred, which should – and will more effectually humble it in public estimation. It was said, that in France, it took a long series of years to raise medicine from the paltriness to which the powerful satire of Moliere laughed it; but how much greater reason have the British public to dread and detest a science, which in its abominations, has trampled morality, religion, and every feeling of common humanity under foot, which has countenanced a tragedy to which the fiction of Bluebeard in his bloody chamber, is but a foil, – and which now unblushingly comes forward to defend on the plea of the advancement of knowledge, the perpetration of cold-blooded murders. Faugh![6]

The 'Shepherd' character (based on James Hogg) in the 'Noctes' of August 1830 takes on the presumed public bias against surgeons and anatomists. He exclaims, 'I ken na amang our poets the match o' my freen Mr Moir o' Musselburgh, surgeon though he be, – and fearsome to think o'! in the way o' his profession, during his college days doobtless a dissector o' dead bodies!' North comes to Moir's rescue: 'But not of him – "gentle lover of nature," – could it be said, as some that shall now be nameless, in the language of Wordsworth, – "We *murder* to dissect!"' Despite concurring in acknowledgement of Moir's 'genius and humanity', the Shepherd remains humorously sceptical and picks up on North's citation of Wordsworth, commenting that while Moir 'wou'd na, gin he cou'd help it, brush the gold or silver dust aff the wings o' a butterflee' he might bring himself 'to shy his beaver at it, for the sake o' sceence'.[7]

As Caroline McCracken-Flesher has recently argued, '[i]n 1827, Robert Knox represented the "march of intellect" in Edinburgh', and when the anatomy murders came to light, 'Edinburgh learned that systematic medicine based on experiment and exploration depended on Burke and Hare.'[8] Her wide-ranging examination of the legacy of the Burke and Hare story in Scottish literature emphasises the un-tellability of their tale and its endurance as a national metaphor of cultural trauma, with each attempt to frame the story resulting in the exposure of new anxieties rather than closure. This chapter examines the construction of Moir as a literary surgeon, by himself and others, as a key component of a counter-discourse – a redemptive medical humanism – that began to take shape before the atrocities of Burke and Hare were known, but which draws upon eighteenth-century Scottish medical culture to re-envision a medical tradition based upon the very 'morality, religion, and every feeling of common humanity' that Knox's murderous 'advancement of knowledge' is said to have 'trampled' underfoot.[9]

While Knox provided a focal point for the 'Noctes', as representing the current errors of the medical profession, Moir's medico-literary project responded more generally to a contemporary popular view of the physician or surgeon as irreligious, immoral, and even inhumane. This was the era that produced Dr Frankenstein, whose loss of humanity was 'emblematic' of the fears of his day.[10] Fatalism and materialism became increasingly associated with the medical profession in the popular imagination.[11] Ruth Richardson outlines the conflict between traditional religious or folkloric valuations of the corpse as an 'object of veneration' and the detached view of the surgeon or anatomist, which enabled the violation of cultural taboos in the name of scientific and medical progress.[12] *Blackwood's*, however, provided a powerful ideological context for the early formation of a counter-discourse, with its longstanding critique of the 'march of intellect' associated with the sceptical philosophers of the Scottish Enlightenment and their heirs in the *Edinburgh Review*. If *Blackwood's* Romantic ideology of cultural nationalism depended upon 'division as its empirical foundation', its construction of idealised medico-literary figures was similarly predicated upon growing cultural divisions.[13]

Literature and Medicine in Scotland

The bifurcation of literary and scientific/medical spheres is traditionally said to have begun in the Romantic era.[14] Scotland enjoyed a strong tradition of literary medical men in the seventeenth and eighteenth centuries, and the physician as a 'man of letters' held a high cultural currency during the Scottish Enlightenment. As Adam Budd has recently argued, prominent medico-literary figures such as the Edinburgh-trained didactic medical poet John Armstrong (1708/9–79) used their literary talents to gain public esteem in the medical marketplace, where 'canny self-promotion' rather than professional efficacy was key.[15] Dorothy Porter and Roy Porter similarly note that Georgian physicians did not achieve fame generally through 'advances in medical science or . . . spectacular breakthroughs in therapeutics', but rather through social visibility; medical power derived less from 'statutory authority' than from celebrity.[16] They cite the Scriblerian satirist John Arbuthnot (*bap.* 1667–*d.* 1735) and the poets Samuel Garth (1660/1–1719) and Mark Akenside (1721–71) as examples of physicians who 'made their mark upon the metropolitan scene' in London.[17] The vibrant club culture of Enlightenment Scotland, including the scholarly societies fostered by the medical schools, where an interest in rhetoric, literature, philosophy and other polite arts was to be deemed essential to a gentleman physician's education, provided another arena for the generation of esteem. John Gregory's *Observations on the Duties and Offices of a Physician and on*

Methods of Prosecuting Enquiries in Philosophy (1770), later revised and republished as *Lectures on the Duties and Qualifications of a Physician* (1772), articulated a particularly enduring defence of the value of medicine as a 'liberal profession'.[18] Proficiency in Latin, Greek and French, familiarity with the history of medicine and natural philosophy, and a general 'knowledge of the world, of men, and of manners', 'though not absolutely necessary to the successful practice of medicine', are considered by Gregory to be 'such ornamental acquisitions, as no physician who has had a regular education is found without'.[19] Gregory's own contribution to polite letters, the moral sentimental guide *A Father's Legacy to his Daughters*, was published posthumously in 1774.

While Gregory's lectures remained a major touchstone through the early nineteenth century in discussions surrounding the reform of medical education, some began to doubt the value of such 'ornamental acquisitions', preferring instead knowledge of modern languages and practical anatomical and clinical training as more favourable to the advancement of medical knowledge. Andrew Duncan, junior, writing in the *Edinburgh Medical and Surgical Journal* in 1827, emphasises the importance of recognising the 'distinction between those kinds of literary and scientific knowledge, which are absolutely indispensable to the safe exercise of the profession; those which it is desirable and for the interest of the practitioner that he should possess, and those which are merely ornamental', and contends that, ultimately, '[m]edicine is a practical profession'.[20] He particularly argues against moves to require a preliminary classical education before the commencement of medical training:

> We are also told that physicians and surgeons, in consequence of an extended preliminary education, are to become not only wiser, but better. . . . All this is very well said; but a great deal more is necessary to attain the wished-for end than compelling every physician to read Greek and be an adept in philosophy.[21]

For Duncan, such classical and philosophical learning was associated with the English universities (i.e. Oxford and Cambridge) rather than with Scottish medical degrees, in which practical knowledge was instead emphasised.[22] Indeed, it was the non-denominational, relatively affordable, and practice-based nature of the Edinburgh medical school that had made it such a popular choice for medical students in the eighteenth century.[23] In the nineteenth century, the increasing knowledge of the structure and function of the body, fuelled by the new pathological anatomy, indicated to many that medical and surgical education should be more scientific.[24]

Further, the traditional medical hierarchy, which had placed the liberally-educated physician in the highest social position, was progressively breaking down at this point. The new regulations for Licentiates of the Royal College of Surgeons in Edinburgh drawn up in 1808 noted the importance of a liberal education for surgeons, in a substantive move towards raising the social status of a profession previously viewed as a manual trade; some prominent surgeons, such as John Thomson, wished to carry that momentum forward.[25] Historians of medicine generally agree that this process was less strained in Scotland, where medical students and surgical apprentices had received training in anatomy together in university and extramural lectures from as early as 1739.[26] Edinburgh surgeons were, in effect, what would come to be known as 'general practitioners' in the early nineteenth century: a class of medical practitioners, according to Irvine Loudon's seminal study, 'created by a public demand for a reliable, education [sic] all-rounder' who was also affordable to the middling classes.[27] Loudon notes that while the upper classes might still turn to the physician, 'the middle ground was occupied fairly and squarely by the general practitioner, and it was a ground embracing more than is usually understood by definitions of the middle classes, since it ranged from domestic servants and labourers to the minor gentry and professional people'.[28] This was the audience base to which Scottish surgeons such as Macnish and Moir needed to appeal, and for which, as this chapter will show in regard to Moir, 'literary' pursuits were no longer necessarily advantageous in promoting one's reputation.

The Scottish tradition of the physician as 'man of letters' was, however, certainly not extinguished at the turn of the century. While the professional standing of the physician, poet and chair of moral philosophy at the University of Edinburgh, Thomas Brown, appears to have been damaged by his poetic pursuits, Andrew Duncan senior successfully cultivated a popular reputation as a convivial medical poet, derived from the boisterous sociability of Enlightenment club culture.[29] He founded the Aesculapian Society in 1773 and the

Harveian Society in 1782, which was intended 'to commemorate the discovery of the circulation of the blood by circulation of the glass'.[30] According to Duncan, occasional '*poetical effusions*' greatly 'added to the hilarity of the convivial meetings of medical men at Edinburgh', and he published a selection of this poetry in 1818, adjoined to his Harveian oration in honour of Alexander Monro, *secundus*, 'to demonstrate to the world, that, although the Medical Practitioners in Edinburgh have not been exempted from quarrels, highly disgraceful to the profession, yet that many of them have lived, do now live, and I trust will continue to live, on the most social and friendly terms with each other'.[31] Duncan senior was one of the most prominent physicians in Edinburgh; according to Henry Cockburn, he appeared 'to live and be happy, and get liked, by . . . mere absurdities'.[32] A young provincial surgeon and budding poet and prose essayist such as Moir was far more uncertain of enjoying a positive reception in both the literary and the medical marketplaces.

Beginning in *Blackwood's*

While today Moir is remembered as a core member of the 'Blackwood group' of writers and as an imitator of John Galt (1779–1839) in *The Life of Mansie Wauch, Tailor in Dalkeith* (1828), during his own lifetime he gained popular renown not only as a sentimental poet, humorist, and lecturer on poetical literature, but also as a medical historian, a devoted provincial surgeon and an outspoken 'contagionist' during the cholera epidemic of 1832.[33] He stands out among the medical contributors to *Blackwood's* in its early years for the sheer breadth of his contribution to literature and medicine and for his eventual prominence as a figure representative of their compatibility. If Macnish at the end of his life is portrayed as concluding that his 'pursuits in the region of fancy' were 'unprofitable' in light of 'the superiority of the principles of science', Moir appears steadfast in his dedication to both spheres.[34] As William Findlay eulogises in 1898, '[h]e is, indeed, one of the solitary examples, not only of the compatibility of medicine with letters, but of their entirely successful union in his own remarkable person'.[35] However, his early attempts to establish himself as a man of letters were marked with trepidation.

Moir's extant correspondence with William Blackwood does not commence until May 1820, and by this point he had acted as partner to the surgeon Thomas Brown for three years in his Musselburgh practice.[36] His early letters express deep concerns regarding the protection of his fledgling reputation as a provincial surgeon from the scandal of becoming known as a literary man. In July 1820 he writes:

> I must decline giving you my name for several reasons – the principal of which is that being actively engaged in <u>proffessional</u> [sic] pursuits, and surrounded by people, who are not of the most liberal tempers, it becomes a matter of necessity that I should not be suspected of <u>literary</u> pursuits.[37]

Blackwood was apparently insistent, and Moir further explains in August 1820:

> You are anxious for my name? – This could not possibly be of any actual service to you, or the Magazine, as I am almost unknown by name in the literary world, and might be highly disadvantageous to me, being much taken up by my proffessional [sic] pursuits, and daily in the company of many, who though elevated in station, and otherwise liberal, cannot be imagined to have much sympathy for dabblers in literature.[38]

Moir's fears were not unwarranted. In his *Autobiographical Recollections* (1874), J. F. Clarke confirms that '[t]here can be no doubt that if a reputation is acquired by a Physician for anything not strictly Medical, it may interfere with his Professional progress', and as discussed above, Macnish had similar qualms.[39] However, if contributing to *Blackwood's* was inherently risky, their eagerness to do so indicates that it also had utility for medical contributors. For Moir, the magazine provided a powerful ideological context for his early considerations of the value of the medical practitioner's involvement in wider literary culture.

'Why Are Professional Men Indifferent Poets?'

The irony of Moir's prose essay, 'Why Are Professional Men Indifferent Poets?', printed anonymously in the January 1821 number of *Blackwood's* (an issue containing four poems by Delta, as well as an anonymous poetic prose essay, 'Flores Poetici'), may have been lost to all but Blackwood himself, who had been made privy to Delta's true identity by October 1820, but the essay takes its meaning from its embedded context within the magazine.[40] An extended study of the 'deadening influence' of '[p]rofessional avocations ... on the finer sensibilities of the mind', it is particularly adamant regarding the medical profession:

> Can it for a moment be supposed that a physician, one whose business it is to be acquainted with the weaknesses and miserable diseases to which our bodies are subject; that one whose daily occupation is the inspection of loathsome sores, and putrifying ulcers, could, in despite of his own observation, preserve in the penetralia of his mind, a noble and unblemished image of human beauty; or that the anatomist, who has glutted over the debasing and repellent horrors of a dissecting table, where the severed limbs of his fellow creatures, 'the secrets of the grave,' are displayed in hideous deformity, to satisfy the hyæna lust of knowledge, could look upon a female face with the rapture, which the mind that conceived Shakespeare's Juliet must have done; or with that sense of angelic delicacy, which must have penetrated the mind of Spenser, ere he conceived the glorious idea of 'Heavenly Una, with her milk-white lamb?'[41]

Moir assumes the same basic premise as Lockhart's infamous attack on John Keats in the 'Cockney School of Poetry' series in August 1818. Lockhart had declared that the young man had talent enough for a 'useful profession', referred to his apprenticeship to 'a worthy apothecary', and lamented that he had fallen prey to the 'poetical mania' of the age.[42] His critique of Keats, whose 'Endymion is not a Greek shepherd, loved by a Grecian goddess' but 'merely a young Cockney rhymester, dreaming a phantastic dream at the full of the moon', is predicated upon the assumption that an apothecary – the very lowest profession within the medical hierarchy – who trades in '"plasters, pills, and ointment boxes"', would be presumptuous to think that he might achieve the glorious ideals of the poetic imagination.[43] According to Lockhart, Keats's poetry is instead vulgarly amorous, as well as politically seditious.[44] However, Moir aims his critique not at the failures of medical (or 'pharmacopolitical') poets themselves, but rather at the present age's valuation of professional life – of '[c]ounting-houses and ledgers', 'of every-day experience, of sickness, dullness, and formality' – over 'generosity, romance, and chivalry': a valuation detrimental to young men of genius.[45] While not necessarily exonerating Keats's poetic genius, he turns the critique back upon modern society and seeks to establish a position for medical poets within its unfavourable conditions.

Referring to Hazlitt's 'Lectures on English Poetry', delivered at the Surrey Institution in 1818, Moir declares: 'We believe that Hazlitt is the first who has told us in definite terms, that as the boundaries of science are enlarged, the empire of imagination is diminished.'[46] This stadial opposition of imagination and science – and an accompanying defence of the religious value of the primitive poetic imagination – reoccurs throughout Moir's corpus and in *Blackwood's* more widely.[47] As Lockhart declares in his 'Remarks on Schlegel's History of Literature' in August 1818:

> We may rave about political economy and chemistry, and despise, if we choose, the simple ages which were more occupied with art than with science, with feeling than with analysing; but to those who consider this world as a preparatory scene, and our earthly life as a school for our intellect, and man as an immortal creature, whose desires and aspirations are at all times after the infinite, the spectacle of this, our boasted age, may perhaps appear to partake at least as much of the humiliating as of the cheering.[48]

Likewise Moir's essay acknowledges what is lost in the reign of scientific and utilitarian values. In this world wherein 'the physician measures out his kindness and attentions at the direct ratio of his expectation of being repaid' and '[m]an, "with the human face divine," is not considered so much as a Being of majestic attributes, and an immortal destiny, but as being of a few days, and full of trouble, a petty insignificant creature, full of fraud and deceit, and selfishness, and subject to an infinite variety of diseases and infirmities', Moir asks:

> How is it to be supposed then, that the men who are continually exposed to the withering influence of these current maxims, and who, to preserve unanimity, are obliged to echo them back, and to concur in their infallibility – how is it to be supposed, that they are to throw off the load that oppresses them – to forget what they hear every day – and

to shut their eyes to every thing that is passing around them – and, in despite of their contracted and desolate view of human nature, and the external world, form a bower of happiness for themselves, in the paradise of imagination?[49]

For Moir, the answer to this question was a continued devotion to his poetical practice. In an article the following year in Constable's *Edinburgh Magazine*, under the pseudonym 'M', he writes of his associates chastising him for the time he spends 'castle-building' and writing poetry, but defends the utility of these extra-professional activities for the sake of 'happiness' and also their generally virtuous nature – their ability to 'banish from the mind the darker and malignant passions, and to replace them with noble emotions, and domestic and benevolent affections!'[50]

'On Vulgar Prejudices Against Literature'

In his anonymous article, 'On Vulgar Prejudices Against Literature', published in *Blackwood's* in May 1821, Moir gives his harshest appraisal of the popular attitudes towards literary medical practitioners. He explains:

> If the scandal of literature is attached to any one's name, it is downright murder committed on his reputation and interest; and if temporal advancement and worldly success depend on his professional efforts, the veriest dunce, and the most ignorant pretender, have a greater chance of success. . . . Akenside attracted neither respect nor admiration in his native town, while his reputation as a poet was a barrier, which all the strenuous efforts he made in his professional career, were insufficient to overcome. Armstrong shared the same fate. . . . Darwin, with more unpoetical prudence, concealed his studies till his medical reputation was established.[51]

This reading of the eighteenth-century physician-writer affords a stark contrast to the arguments of critics such as Marie Mulvey Roberts and Roy Porter, who point to the eighteenth century as the heyday of the physician-writer – a period in which '[w]riter-physicians like Erasmus Darwin did not associate themselves with a single professional identity nor . . . see their writing subjected to a textual discrimination which divorced literature from medicine'.[52] While Moir may be retrospectively diagnosing past writers with his own anxieties, Anne Seward's biography of Darwin, published in 1804, appears to be the source of his comments regarding Darwin, Armstrong, and Akenside.[53]

Regardless of the accuracy of the matter, Moir successfully yokes his critique of the 'vulgar prejudice' against the literary medical practitioner to what David Higgins has identified as the wider Blackwoodian and later Fraserian defence of great literary genius. According to Higgins, in both magazines literary genius was defended against perceived associations with moral transgression as well as the encroaching threat of Benthamite utilitarianism, which represented the creative arts as 'no more than amusing luxuries'.[54] In this context Moir affirms the unique ability of literary studies to elevate the soul, enabling the achievement of a 'powerful generalization of thought', 'masterly command over the feelings', and that 'unbounded range of imagination', which 'constitutes [man's] excellency among the order of being'.[55] Moir laments: 'Strange, that the essence and fountain of all moral rectitude, and political improvement, should be polluted with the venom of envy!'[56] Further, building upon the Blackwoodian valuation of Schlegel's national literary history, Moir glorifies the importance of literature in capturing the genius of a nation (or, one might add, a profession) for future generations.[57] He does see the perceived value of literature as improving in recent years, as now 'the first walks in the learned professions are filled by men, eminent for their literature', but he notes that there are still many who 'glory in being acquainted only with the one thing needful'. Such persons are viewed as inhibiting progress, as '[t]hey are like horses yoked in a mill, that plod round, and round, and round, until they are tired; and "as the morning saw, the evening sees"'.[58] As we will see, this is the same line of reasoning that Moir will use to defend the importance of the history of medicine.

In the 'Noctes' of August 1830, Delta's insistence that 'the study of elegant literature' strengthens both 'the moral and intellectual energies' of his surgical practice is clearly a more overt and publicly identifiable statement of the discourses he himself had propagated anonymously in the early 1820s. This construction positions him as a unifying figure for the 'severed faculties of reason and sentiment' within the specialised context of Scottish medicine – evidencing the productive compatibility of the literary and healing arts at a point when the reputation of the medical profession was most certainly not for sentiment.[59] However, if North's celebration of Moir places him in a long line of medical poets – 'Garth, Armstrong, Arbuthnot, Akenside, Glyn, and many other men of poetical powers, or otherwise fine genius' – who have adorned the profession 'with the flowers of literature',[60] Moir himself turned to the history of medicine to shape his medico-literary identity and to argue that the study of the history of medicine, and relatedly, philosophy and the classics, would provide a moral and religious basis for the advancement of medical knowledge.

The Ancient History of Medicine

According to Moir's letters to Blackwood, his primary motivation in writing *Outlines of the Ancient History of Medicine* was the promotion of his own medical reputation by providing evidence to the wider public that he could turn his 'attention to other things than light literature'.[61] The idea of the history was first suggested to Moir by Galt, celebrated for his fictional 'conjectural' histories serialised in *Blackwood's*.[62] On 4 September 1830 Galt wrote to inform Moir that he had spoken to the London publisher Henry Colburn, who 'thinks one volume on the History of Medicine will do very well'.[63] However, by his letter of 21 September, it had transpired that Colburn's associate, Richard Bentley, had already spoken to Dr William Hamilton and invited him to compose a history of medicine to be published by Colburn and Bentley.[64] Undeterred, Moir turned to Blackwood as a potential publisher, and by the end of January 1831, he notes that his manuscript is 'so far advanced that it might be put to press quam primum having only three chapters to write'.[65] Blackwood did take some convincing, and Moir assured him 'that a work on Medical History is wanted in English' and 'so far as the history of practical medicine is concerned we have the whole field to ourselves'.[66] He also called upon Blackwood's personal obligations to him: 'In a Proffessional [sic] point of view I am aware that it is necessary for me to produce some treatise of this kind, and I am sure you will do what you can to farther my prospects in life.'[67]

Moir's decision to turn to the history of medicine may have been informed by its key role in establishing the authority of the medical profession in early nineteenth-century Britain. Through the eighteenth century, many medical texts began with a history of medicine, but despite Moir's claims to his text's singularity, as James Allard has evidenced, 'several dedicated histories of medicine appeared throughout the eighteenth and early nineteenth centuries that point to the field's desire to tell its own story, in its own words, to serve its own interests'.[68] Allard points to John Aikin's *Biographical Memoirs of Medicine in Great Britain From the Revival of Literature to the Time of Harvey* (1780) and Benjamin Hutchinson's *Biographia Medica* (1799) as examples which take the form of biographies, noting the importance of individual medical geniuses to Romantic medicine, while citing Hamilton's *The History of Medicine* (1831) and Richard Walker's *Memoirs of Medicine* (1799) as exemplifying a wider approach. As Frank Huisman and John Harley Warner explain, this was a pivotal period for the development of medical historiography in which the new historical consciousness, particularly prominent in Germany, led physician-historians such as Kurt Sprengel (1766–1833), who is often heralded as the 'founding father of modern medical history', to move beyond the focus on biography and bibliography and to instead examine the evolution of medical thought, 'presupposing links between medicine, philosophy, and general culture'.[69]

In the context of post-Enlightenment Scotland, the study of history was viewed as another aspect of the 'Science of Man', and the relationship between the progress of medical theory and practice and philosophy had been a major preoccupation of Scottish Enlightenment physicians.[70] As Michael Barfoot has noted, Cullen provided historical narratives at the commencement of his courses on the practice of physic and chemistry, 'similar in form to the conjectural or theoretical history, much loved by the Scots in general'.[71] These historical narratives provided a vital part of his medical teaching based on philosophical system and illustrated that medical progress was dependent upon 'the state of refinement in society, and, in particular, on the prevailing "ardour in the culture of philosophy"'.[72] Moir's history participates in this philosophical and cultural turn, exposing how each era's dominant belief systems shape, or limit, the progress of medicine.

History and Anatomy

Unsurprisingly for a medical history written at the height of the anatomy debates, a key villain in Moir's narrative is the popular prejudice against human dissection. He points to the period in which Alexandria rose as a great seat of learning, as when 'that popular prejudice first relaxed, in allowing the examination of dead bodies, – a triumph of the most singular kind for the furtherance of medicine; the ignorance of human anatomy being a perpetual stumbling-block in the path of its professors'.[73] While Moir associated the anatomical horrors of Herophilus, who was accused by 'Celsus, Tertullian, and others' of 'the shocking barbarity of opening the bodies of living criminals for the furtherance of their physiological views' with the immorality of Knox in his letter to Macnish, here he ascribes these accusations to 'the horror with which human dissection was at first regarded, acquiring its utmost popular exaggeration'.[74]

Moir had previously explored this 'popular exaggeration' through his most famous Blackwoodian character, 'Mansie Wauch'. The first 'Wonderful Passage in the Life of Mansie Wauch, Tailor', which appeared in *Blackwood's* in October 1824, relates Mansie's trials standing guard in a graveyard to prevent the 'resurrection-men' from 'howking up the bodies from their damp graves, and harling them away to the College'.[75] Mansie laments:

> Tell me that doctors and graduates maun ha'e the dead; but tell it not to Mansie Wauch, that our hearts maun be trampled in the mire of scorn, and our best feelings laughed at, in order that a bruise may be properly plaistered up, or a sair head cured. Verily, the remedy is waur than the disease.[76]

The critique continues later in the series when Mansie and his wife, 'Nanse', discuss their son's professional prospects. Nanse suggests that he become a doctor, which prompts Mansie to list the horrors daily encountered by medical men,

> to say naething of rampaging wi' dark lanterns, and double-tweel dreadnoughts, aboot gousty kirk-yards, amang humlock and lang nettles, the haill night ower, like spunkie – shoving the dead corpses, winging-sheets and a', into cornsacks, and boiling their banes, after they have dissectit a' the red flesh aff them, into a big cauldron, to get out the marrow to mak' drogs of.[77]

According to Mansie, no amount of monetary remuneration can 'mak up for the loss of a man's having a' his feelings seared to iron, and his soul made into whunstane, yea, into the nether-millstane, by being airt and pairt in sic dark and devilish abominations'.[78]

As Tim Marshall has argued, the 'anatomy literature' of this period, and particularly Shelley's *Frankenstein*, at times portrays the horrors of grave-robbing in order to convince the public of the need for legislation which would provide surgeons with a regular supply of unclaimed bodies from the country's pauper workhouses and thereby put the resurrectionists out of business. Such legislation was seen as vital to establish the dignity of the profession.[79] Both 'Mansie Wauch' and *Outlines of the Ancient History of Medicine* contribute to this agenda, but rather by gently satirising popular aversion and evidencing the necessity of anatomical study for the advancement of medical knowledge. The latter was also the line taken in the anonymous novel *Murderers of the Close* (1829), which, as Lisa Rosner indicates, worked to exonerate Knox and jarringly included a direct statement on the necessity of anatomical study in the middle of a sensational tale.[80] Similarly, the *New Monthly Magazine* explicitly advertised the tale 'The Victim. By A Medical Student' in 1831 as promoting the anatomy legislation, while Gooch recommended William MacMichael's *The Golden-Headed Cane* (1827), 'a modest little volume, containing sketches of the lives and manners of our most eminent physicians', to evidence 'the absolute necessity of a thorough anatomical education, even for those medical men who have nothing to do with the practice of surgery'.[81] However, in 'Mansie Wauch' Moir also participates in a wider Blackwoodian discourse, forwarded, for example, in Wilson's pious sentimental fiction, which esteemed the morality and religious devotion of the Scottish peasantry and idealised them as standing outside the individualist 'march of intellect'. For Moir the dignity of the profession rested not only upon an end to the resurrectionists' trade, but also upon a system of medical education which might produce physicians and surgeons with similarly well-regulated moral and religious sentiments, and in this he built upon a long Scottish tradition which considered moral virtue as key to the development of medical science – a tradition itself in need of resurrection in the popular imagination following the atrocities of Burke and Hare.[82]

Medical Education and Morality

One of Moir's 'most cordial friends', John Abercrombie, published his popular medico-philosophical guide, *Inquiries Concerning the Intellectual Powers and the Investigation of Truth* (1830), just one year prior to Moir's history.[83] Participating in the reaction against Humean sceptical philosophy led by Reid and Stewart, Abercrombie appealed to the divine first cause as the basis for all natural law and viewed medical practice as providing insight into 'the power and wisdom of the Eternal One'.[84] The text went through at least sixteen editions by 1860 and was directed as a guide to 'the younger members of the medical profession'.[85] It contains a final section on the 'well-regulated mind', which necessitated not only reason and judgement, but also 'a sound condition of the moral feelings'.[86] According to Abercrombie, '[a] reasonable man is one who, both in the formation of his opinions and the regulation of his conduct, gives the due weight and influence to all facts and considerations which ought to influence his decision'.[87] Those of an opposite character are either inconsistent in their opinions and conduct, 'led away by hasty impressions, or feeble and inadequate motives', or tenaciously adherent to false principles, despite having framed opinions on inadequate grounds.[88] The latter tendency is associated with those who deny 'the existence of a great first cause', as well as those who allow 'personal feeling or emotion' to control their judgement, as '[i]t is thus that a vitiated and depraved state of the moral feelings at last misleads the judgment'.[89] While Abercrombie also writes of the dangers of the imagination, uncontrolled by reason, as such a mind 'is not disposed to examine, with any careful minuteness, the real condition of things' but is rather 'content with ignorance, because environed with something more delicious than knowledge, in the paradise which imagination creates', he also regards 'that view of man, which regards his understanding alone' as '[c]old and contracted':

> The highest state of man consists in his purity as a moral being; and in the habitual culture and full operation of those principles, by which he looks forth to others scenes and other times. Among these are desires and longings, which nought in earthly science can satisfy; which soar beyond the sphere of sensible things, and find no object worthy of their capacities, until, in humble adoration, they rest in the contemplation of God.[90]

In his life of Macnish, Moir declares Abercrombie to be 'destined to exert no inconsiderable influence, not only over the progress of medical science, but over the intellect and moral feelings of succeeding generations'.[91]

In his attempt to trace the rules by which the intellectual and moral powers of medical enquirers should be guided, Abercrombie enters into the longstanding Scottish debate regarding the value of philosophy in guiding medical practice.[92] A review of his text published in the *Edinburgh Medical and Surgical Journal* neatly characterises those 'practical persons' against whom Abercrombie was writing at this time:

> Every thing which has the air of philosophy they represent as not only useless but pernicious to the genuine physician, by diverting his attention from the business of his profession, and by unfitting him for those prompt and practical applications of his knowledge which are indispensable to the successful exercise of the art. By such persons an invidious line is drawn between theory and practice, the object of which is to throw a degree of discredit and contempt, not only on all the theoretical branches of medical knowledge, but on all those collateral sciences, in which it is pretended it is impossible to recognize any practical application of the healing art.[93]

A reviewer of Moir's text for the *Edinburgh Literary Journal* similarly praises Moir for illustrating 'how far he is above those narrow-minded empirics who think practice incompatible with theory'.[94] While Moir illustrates how philosophical speculations throughout the ages perverted the course of medicine, according to his history, it is philosophy that raises medicine 'to the dignity of a science'.[95] He identifies 'Pythagoras and his disciples' as the first 'to rise over the shadows into the sunlight of truth', and to speculate 'from effects as to their causes' and draw 'inferences, sometimes indeed unsatisfactory, but always ingenious'.[96]

Like Abercrombie, Moir also saw his text as most relevant for the rising generation. According to his letter to Blackwood in January 1831, he was particularly keen to market the work to the medical students of Edinburgh and was eager to have the text in print 'before the end of April, when the Medical classes rise'.[97] In the lead up to the rising of medical classes the following year, Moir published a letter 'To the Students of Medicine' in *Fraser's Magazine*, which covertly advertises the importance of his history. Macnish praises his friend's Fraserian letter, writing that '[i]t hits hard, but justly, and will tell with good effect upon the shoulders of the sumphs'.[98]

The letter, addressed to 'Mr. Yorke', the Fraserian equivalent of Christopher North, is a reworking of an article Moir first intended for *Blackwood's*. However, Blackwood refused the article on the grounds that 'though excellent it does not quite come up to what Christopher would find it necessary to say & dilate upon were he to take up so important a subject'.[99] In January 1830 Moir requested the piece be returned to be published in two parts as 'On Medical Literature and Education' within the *Edinburgh Literary Gazette*.[100] Both this and the Fraserian version trace the current defects in medical literature to medical education, and in particular, 'the deficiency of a preparatory classical education'.[101] In the Fraserian version, he links his critique to the magazine's wider deprecation of literary mediocrity,[102] opening with the declaration, 'WHETHER or not a reformer in politics, there can be no doubt that you are one in literature,' and explaining that 'our medical treatises are still deformed by that quackery in disguise, as to matter, and that unclassical, rude, and plebeian coarseness, as to manner, which evince a radical defect somewhere'.[103] Within the *Edinburgh Literary Gazette*, Moir's articles carry on from a review of a medico-popular text that is used as a springboard to deprecate medical men as 'pedants' who write unreadable books and raise 'horror and hue-and-cry . . . whenever a volume issues from the press with anything like an extra-medical stamp upon it, or which may be thought to profane the hieroglyphic arcana of the science'.[104] One might speculate that what 'Christopher would find it necessary to say' is said months later in the 'Noctes' of August 1830; however, Moir's letter, as it appears in *Fraser's*, builds upon his own previous contributions to *Blackwood's*, while also endorsing his history.

In his letter Moir describes the young medical student, overwhelmed by the heterodoxy of current opinions:

> Yesterday he was told, that in mercury and its chemical combinations may be found specifics for all the diseases that eloped from Pandora's box; and to-day he learns, from perhaps the same authority, that half the ailments afflicting modern society arise from their indiscriminate exhibition.[105]

The blame for this dismal state of affairs is laid squarely at the feet of 'medical men themselves, and not in their calling', as '[t]he experience of a long-linked succession of ages . . . ought to have led to a very different result'.[106] As he does in his history, Moir considers diseases to 'remain specifically and intrinsically the same'. It is 'only, the self-will of every generation of Esculapians' which 'goads them on to the independency of looking upon them with other eyes than those of their ancestors'. As such, 'they erect an idol each for themselves, which the succeeding generations, each for itself, calcitrates and heels over'.[107] An attention to history is affirmed as necessary for true collective, organic progress, and in his 'Preface' to his medical history, Moir echoes his Blackwoodian essay of 1821, warning that without it, 'like the mill-horse, we may work in a circle, tread the same ground over and over again, and, without progressing, leave matters just as we found them'.[108]

Moir's critique was expressed in the conservative medical periodical press at this time, albeit in more subdued terms. In a letter 'To the Editor of the London Medical Gazette' in November 1829, one contributor notes the editorial time that might be saved if knowledge of medical history prevented contributors from sending 'the "results of observations" made and recorded before they were born'.[109] The letter is humorously signed, after the protagonist of Walter Scott's novel *The Antiquary*, 'Jonathan Oldbuck. Monkbarns, Nov. 1, A. D. 1829'. A flattering review of Moir's history, also in the *London Medical Gazette,* presents his text as a solution to this prevailing problem and muses:

> It has often been to us matter of much surprise that, among all the various suggestions offered of late years for the improvement of medical education, no notice has been taken of the great advantage that might be derived from the study of medical history.[110]

Moir's letter 'To the Students of Medicine' particularly engages with this pervasive debate regarding the reform of medical education.

In establishing his recommendations for ameliorating what he deems to be the dire state of contemporary medical education, Moir references the 'pamphleteering war' in Edinburgh between 'Dr. Duncan and Dr. John Thompson [sic], Dr. Craigie, Dr. Robertson, Dr. Abercrombie, and a host of red-hot auxiliaries on either side, as to whether a preliminary classical education was necessary for a medical practitioner'.[111] This debate was spurred on by the Royal Commission of Inquiry into the State of the Universities of Scotland, which was established in 1826 by Robert Peel and published its report in 1830. One result of the report was a recommendation that medical candidates be required to take a preliminary examination on their classical knowledge before being allowed to matriculate into the medical faculty.[112] According to Rosner's analysis, the Scottish universities systematically ignored the report and got away with it, since 'Parliament, caught up in reforming itself in the 1830s, was too busy to get back to the Scottish Universities until 1858.'[113] As Rosner indicates, '[t]he idea that a physician must be a liberally-educated gentleman to practice among gentlemen was hardly new' and was, in fact, part of a Scottish tradition stemming back to Gregory; however, the dismissive response of the medical faculties at this time indicates a turn away from classical authors in favour of the ever-expanding modern medical periodical press.[114]

Moir clearly comes out on the side of those such as Abercrombie, who argued that a liberal education, which enabled one to develop 'a mind well trained to habits of correct reasoning, and philosophical inquiry', was necessary before beginning a medical degree.[115] Further, in line with John Thomson's concurrent campaign to raise the status of the profession through further educational reform, in his Fraserian letter Moir also confirms the necessity of a liberal education for surgical apprentices.[116] According to Moir the vast majority of students, overwhelmed by the freedom of their situation, soon find that 'the dismemberment of a rotten subject at Mr. Pattison's or Mr. Partridge's' has no chance against 'the savoury dissection of a stubble goose at the sign of the Bell and the Savage'.[117] Exceptions to this rule fall into two categories: those who have had a preliminary classical education and those with a 'strong uncultivated intellect' who are prone to speculation. Students in the first category have well-established 'moral principles and religious beliefs', and 'in the examination of the structure of the human body, they behold only a wonderful adaptation of means to ends in the scheme of an all-wise Providence'. Students in the latter category, however, are liable to fall prey to fatalism and materialism. Their uncultivated minds have 'a greater zeal after truth than philosophical acumen in discovering it', and they only perceive 'that one age has only pulled down one theory to set up another, whose duration proved not a whit more permanent'. It is at the anatomy table that 'their loosely hanging principles are unsettled, and probably upset forever':

> In the decay of the material frame they think that they behold the utter extinction of man, whose moral and intellectual endowments they have come to regard as only as the result of material organisation. Fatalism, in all its gloom, takes possession of their minds; and many of them have the hardihood to declare in words what Lawrence has promulgated in writing.[118]

The surgeon William Lawrence had inspired a vehement debate regarding the materiality of mind in his lectures at the Royal College of Surgeons of London in 1816. He asserted that 'mind was a function of the brain', and since '[t]he logical corollary of this view was that the mind/soul could not survive physical death . . . Lawrence's theory was immediately vilified as representing an argument for atheism'.[119]

Moir's tale 'The Wounded Spirit', serialised in *Fraser's* between May and November 1830, features a similar reaction to the anatomy table. In the tale the sensitive confessional protagonist, who has elected to study medicine 'because it was a grave, gloomy profession, connected with all that is heart-desolating and mournful', finds anatomical study unbearable.[120] Battling 'the fastidiousness and the squeamish delicacy' of his impressions, he attempts to view the anatomical dissections as 'the details of a noble and generous system', but laments

> I perceived with a compunctuous sorrow, that all my romantic ideas of the constitution of human society, of life, and man, and nature, were passing from me like shutting flowers at nightfall; and that if my mind could not preserve its energy undiminished, I ran imminent risk of subsiding into a misanthropic and gloomy fatalist.[121]

Abercrombie's answer to this risk was a reaffirmation of Paleyan natural theology and pious resignation:

> The medical observer, in an especial manner, has facts at all times before him which are in the highest degree calculated to fix his deep

and serious attention. In the structure and economy of the human body, he has proofs, such as no other branch of natural science can furnish, of the power and wisdom of the Eternal One. Let him resign his mind to the influence of these truths, and learn to rise, in humble adoration: And, familiar as he is with human suffering and death, let him learn to estimate the value of those truths, which have power to heal the broken heart, and to cheer the bed of death with the prospect of immortality.[122]

In this statement Abercrombie builds upon what Lisbeth Haakonssen has termed the 'Edinburgh ideal of the good physician' as forwarded by Gregory, Thomas Percival (1740–1804), and Benjamin Rush (1746–1831).[123] 'Like Hippocrates,' she explains, 'the physician would make his interests subservient to those of his patient and his profession and, as a Christian, subservient to the general good of mankind.'[124] Moir's distinctive contribution to the continuation of this discourse in the nineteenth century was not only his promotion of a liberal education for physicians and surgeons as a means to produce virtuous practitioners, but also his popularisation of this Christian medical ideal through his poetry and, posthumously, through his biographical canonisation.

'Delta': Poet and Moralist

Whether addressing ruined abbeys, the changing seasons or youthful lovers now aged, Moir's poetry consistently turned upon religious themes, reflecting his 'profound veneration for the Church of Scotland'.[125] 'Sabbath. *In Six Sonnets*' perhaps best expresses the piety of Delta. Religion becomes 'SOOTHER of life, physician of all ail, / Thou, more than reputation, wealth, or power, / In the soul's garden the most glorious flower'.[126] The Congregational minister William Lindsay Alexander (1808–84) posthumously praises Moir for his religious and moral feelings, noting that '[i]t is impossible to read his poems, without marking abundant proofs of a deep sensibility to religious impressions, and a strong tendency to moral reflection'.[127] Alexander also alludes to the continuity between Moir's poetic and medical reputations, particularly in the immediate locality of Musselburgh, where you might ask 'the first boy you met' about Moir and receive the reply: '"Him? ou, that's just the doctor; – *Dailta*, ye ken."'[128] As Alexander notes, the statue erected in Moir's honour on the banks of the Esk displays an inscription that celebrates this hybrid identity: Moir was 'beloved as a man, honoured as a citizen, esteemed as a physician, and celebrated as a poet'.[129]

Moir's *Domestic Verses* (1843) was widely considered to contain 'the most exquisite and perfect productions of his muse' and to best evidence his 'forcible moral painting'.[130] The successive deaths of his three infant children in 1838 and 1839 inspired the collection, and according to Moir it was originally intended only for private circulation amongst friends whom he thought might be inclined to view the influence of his family tragedies on his 'heart and imagination'.[131] However, as he explains in a letter to his future biographer Thomas Aird (1802–76), he 'received letters from Wordsworth, Mrs Southey, Lockhart, Trench, Tennyson, White, Warren, Dickens, Montgomery, Whewell, Ferrier, and many others, which left me no grounds for refusing to make my little book a publication'.[132] The 'little book' was published the same year by Blackwood, republished as a new edition in 1871, and was the only collection of Moir's poetry to be published as a centenary edition in 1898. The privately circulated version contains just seven short poems, the first of which, 'To My Infant Daughter – E. C. M.', is a meditation on fatherly hopes and fears, while the remainder are all devoted to his departed children.[133] The pathos of Moir's reflections on the suddenness of his child's death in 'Casa Wappy' is tempered by resignation to the workings of Providence and appeals to the comforts of religion: ''tis sweet balm to our despair, / Fond, fairest boy, / That heaven is God's, and thou are there'.[134] In his memoir of Moir, Aird quotes Jeffrey's praise for the *Domestic Verses* in a letter to the author: 'I cannot resist the impulse of thanking you, with all my heart, for the deep gratification you have afforded me, and the soothing, and, I hope, *bettering* emotions which you have excited.'[135] According to a reviewer in *MacPhail's Edinburgh Ecclesiastical Journal*, these poetic powers were achieved not in spite of Moir's medical career but rather because of it: 'in the course of his daily duty, with the varying aspects of earth, and sea, and sky around him, with his fellow man his constant study, and a home of sweet and hushed affection ever awaiting him, he had just the best school he could have had for the nourishment of these happy gifts'.[136] However, his letters to Blackwood and his sons are also peppered with references to his unremitting life as a country surgeon, which often interrupted his literary pursuits.[137]

From as early as 1829, Blackwood and his sons, along with Abercrombie, aware of the toil of the country practitioner and with 'sanguine hopes of his success in the wider field proposed', repeatedly urged Moir to set up practice in Edinburgh.[138] However, according to his Blackwoodian obituary in 1851, Moir's 'attachment to Musselburgh' and his inability 'to forsake his practice in a locality where the poor had a claim upon him' explain why he, with his 'brilliant prospects', still 'preferred the hard and laborious life of a country practitioner'.[139] His labours became most arduous during the cholera epidemic of 1832, when he became Medical Secretary to the Board of Health at Musselburgh and published two pamphlets arguing for the contagious nature of the disease.[140] This was yet another critical point in Scottish medical history when medical practitioners were vilified *en masse*. As Richardson notes, the need 'to remove poor cholera victims to special hospitals, and to bury the dead swiftly in isolated cholera burial grounds' offended 'the popular desire to defend traditional death observances' and fuelled fears that medical authorities were coercing 'the poor into hospitals for use in vivisection experiments, for dissection after death, or to keep down the population'.[141] Macnish writes to Moir from Glasgow in February 1832:

> The people have a dreadful antipathy to any person being sent to the hospitals. They stupidly imagine that they are murdered (burked!) by the doctors; and, last night, when they were conveying a patient there, they were attacked by the mob.[142]

Moir's life of Macnish details his and his friend's laborious attempts to promote the contagionist theory of disease causation in professional circles and to give advice on disease prevention and treatment to both popular and professional audiences.[143] While his efforts garnered the increased recognition within medical circles that he so desired, his devotion to his local community during the epidemic also became part of his lasting medico-literary legacy.[144] Moir's obituary relates how he spent 'night and day in attendance upon the sufferers', toiling with 'more than the enthusiasm of youth', such that 'the morning' often 'found him watching by the bed of some poor inmate of a cottage whom the arrow of the pestilence had stricken'.[145]

Moir versifies selfless medical morality in his poem 'Hippocrates to the Ambassadors of Artaxerxes', published in the *Edinburgh Literary Gazette* in 1829 and reprinted in *Blackwood's* in 1836. In the poem Hippocrates rejects 'an invitation from Artaxerxes, King of Persia, with a promise of every reward and honour he might desire, provided he would repair to his dominions during a season of pestilence'. After describing his watchful and affectionate service to the impoverished sick of Greece, he instructs the Ambassadors:

> Go – bid your monarch pause, from all apart,
> And ask this question of his conscious heart,
> . . .
> Ask him if these, the pageants of a king,
> Can ever to his thoughts such rapture bring,
> As that I feel, when, as I journey on,
> The pale youth rises from the wayside stone,
> With health-rekindling cheek, and palms outspread,
> To call down bliss on my unworthy head, – [146]

Hippocrates' contentment in his 'cheerful home', his dedication to his 'country, fair and free, / Green Cos, the glory of the Ægean sea', and his valuation of what Moir once termed the 'feeling of common humanity' above monetary gain echo the values attributed to the Scottish peasantry, the 'Mansie Wauchs', in the proto-Kailyard literature popularised in *Blackwood's* in the 1820s.[147]

In turn, his Blackwoodian obituary and numerous reviews of Aird's memoir exalt Moir himself as the type of dedicated country practitioner celebrated by Scott in *The Surgeon's Daughter* (1827) and later in the century by Maclaren in *A Doctor of the Old School* (1895).[148] Some found this exaltation overdrawn. A review in *The New Quarterly Review and Digest of Current Literature* declares:

> If to be a respectable man and a useful surgeon – if to ride twenty miles a
> day, to bleed and bone-set and to sit up at night, to polish graceful inanities

in smoothly-shining rhymes – if to have written 'Mansie Wauch' in prose, and 'the Legend of Genevieve' in verse – if to have epistolised some small toadyism to the most popular of the authors of the day, and to have drawn a pun or two from poor Tom Hood – if these be good title-deeds to exact a perpetual remembrance from posterity – good lack, poor posterity! A thousand of such great men die every year.[149]

However, Moir's dutiful life – 'emphatically dedicated to God and man, and marked by industry, self-denial and usefulness' – was celebrated not just for its medical or literary eminence, but also for its evangelical utility.[150] Biographies and obituaries of diverse professional men, including physicians, were regularly published in religious monthlies, such as the *Wesleyan-Methodist Magazine*, and in 1847 the Religious Tract Society of London, the primary publisher of evangelical tracts, published *Sketches of Eminent Medical Men*.[151] Citing the 'scepticism and infidelity' often associated with the medical profession, an introductory manifesto presents the biographical sketches as evidence 'that there is no necessary connexion between either the studies or the active duties of a medical man, and the denial or practical neglect of those great truths which have been brought to light by the gospel'. The medical profession, 'more than any other', unfolds 'to the eye of the intelligent observer the wonderful works of God'.[152]

As William Christie has recently argued, the common thread of the vast array of scientific articles appearing in the early numbers of *Blackwood's* is their contribution to the magazine's steadfast opposition to the separation between science and religion in the present day, and, as will be discussed in the following chapter, Moir was not alone among his Blackwoodian cohorts in exemplifying an ideal moral and religious medico-literary figure.[153] The same number that featured Delta as a counter to the inhumanity of Knox included the first number of Samuel Warren's popular series *Passages from the Diary of a Late Physician*, which was serialised in the magazine between 1830 and 1837. As with Delta's medico-literary persona, Warren's late physician appeals to the cult of sensibility with evangelical fervour. In his preface to the People's Edition of 1854, Warren writes of his attempt to revitalise the reputation of physicians by reawakening 'society to a sense of its incalculable obligations to Medical Men' and revealing '[t]he amount of misery and suffering which they alleviate, cheerfully and patiently, often altogether gratuitously, and too-frequently with ill-requital – nay, cruel ingratitude'.[154]

If physicians and surgeons were lampooned in a range of media through the eighteenth and early nineteenth centuries – from the satirical novels of Smollett and the popular prints of Hogarth to the horrors of *Frankenstein* and the 'pawky' humour of 'Mansie Wauch' – in Victorian literature 'the Smollettian brute was replaced by the medical man of the highest ideals, if also tragic flaws', such as the examples portrayed in Harriet Martineau's *Deerbrook* (1839), Anthony Trollope's *Dr. Thorne* (1858), and George Eliot's *Middlemarch* (1871–2).[155] Tabitha Sparks follows Lawrence Rothfield in identifying the 'doctor-hero' as a Victorian concept, as 'the rise of professionalism popularized a middle-class realm of subject matter, including the dramas and stories attached to the learned professions'.[156] However, while Sparks notes that 'Romantic and early Victorian doctors were vulnerable to charges of "body snatching"', she and others have not identified the formulation of a redemptive counter-discourse in Scottish letters in the aftermath of the Burke and Hare scandal.[157] This Scottish counter-discourse may be viewed as the bridge between Georgian satire and Victorian idealisation, and the inspiration for what might be called the 'medical kailyard' of Ian Maclaren in the 1890s as well as, earlier in the century, the writings of Dr John Brown (1810–82), author of the sentimental surgical tale 'Rab and his Friends' (1858).[158]

Moir's particular medico-literary endeavours are also credited with the creation of a reading public that could once again value literary medical practitioners. In his memoir Aird gives 'Honour to the "Gold-headed Cane"': 'two of the finest poems on the Daisy, since Chaucer's many exquisite touches of affection for the flower, are by Dr Mason Good and Dr Moir of Musselburgh'. Aird quotes a letter to Moir from William Howitt (1792–1879) praising him for proving 'that medical men may be devoted to their professional duties as well as distinguished in literature, and that there *may be* a public wise enough to see that'.[159] As we will see in the following chapter, Warren's late physician inspired a range of physicians and surgeons to follow his example; however, particularly in the case of Warren's series, medical morality only served to reify the authority of the nineteenth-century medical practitioner.

Notes

1. [John Wilson], 'Noctes Ambrosianæ. No. LI', *BEM*, 28 (August 1830, Part II), 383–436 (p. 418).
2. Robert Macnish to William Blackwood, 10 July 1830, NLS MS 4028, fols 17–18.
3. Ibid.
4. Martin Fido, *Bodysnatchers* (London: Weidenfield & Nicolson, 1988), p. 130, as quoted in Marshall, *Murdering to Dissect*, p. 76.
5. 'Noctes Ambrosianæ. No. XLI', *BEM*, 25 (March 1829), 371–400 (p. 388).
6. Moir, *The Modern Pythagorean*, vol. 1, pp. 123–4.
7. [Wilson], 'Noctes Ambrosianæ. No. LI', p. 386.
8. McCracken-Flesher, *The Doctor Dissected*, p. 56.
9. Moir, *The Modern Pythagorean*, vol. 1, pp. 123–4.
10. Richardson, *Death, Dissection and the Destitute*, p. xvii.
11. Ibid. p. 94. On the associations between the medical profession and fatalism and materialism, see Porter and Porter, *Patient's Progress*, p. 54. Another example may be found in Olinthus Gregory's *Memoirs of the Life, Writings, and Character, Literary, Professional, and Religious, of the Late John Mason Good, M.D.* (London: Henry Fisher, Son, and Co., 1828), wherein he notes: 'It is often asserted, that medical men are more inclined to indifference in religion, and, in fact, to infidelity, than any other class of men' (p. 345).
12. Richardson, *Death, Dissection and the Destitute*, p. 51. See also Rosner, *The Anatomy Murders*, p. 167.
13. Duncan, *Scott's Shadow*, p. 61.
14. For the traditional account, see Roberts and Porter, 'Introduction', in Roberts and Porter (eds), *Literature & Medicine during the Eighteenth Century*, pp. 2–3; Ruston provides a more recent overview in *Creating Romanticism*, pp. 1–27.
15. Budd, *John Armstrong's The Art of Preserving Health*, p. 24.
16. Porter and Porter, *Patient's Progress*, p. 123.
17. Ibid. p. 124.
18. For this cultural formation, see Guerrini, '"A Club of little villains"', in Roberts and Porter (eds), *Literature & Medicine during the Eighteenth Century*, pp. 226–44; Jenkinson, *Scottish Medical Societies, 1731–1939*.
19. McCullough, *John Gregory's Writings on Medical Ethics and Philosophy of Medicine*, p. 98.
20. [Andrew Duncan], 'Medical Education', *EMSJ*, 27 (April 1827), 349–77 (pp. 362–3). This attribution is based on the signature of 'A D Jr'.

21. Ibid. pp. 370–1.
22. Ibid. pp. 375–6.
23. Hamilton, 'The Scottish Enlightenment and Clinical Medicine', p. 107; Haakonssen, *Medicine and Morals in the Enlightenment*, pp. 12–19; Corfield, *Power and the Professions in Britain*, p. 159.
24. Dingwall, *A History of Scottish Medicine*, p. 193.
25. Rosner, *Medical Education in the Age of Improvement*, p. 144. See [Thomson], *Hints Respecting the Improvement of the Literary & Scientific Education of Candidates for the Degree of Doctor of Medicine in the University of Edinburgh.*
26. Rosner, *Medical Education in the Age of Improvement*, p. 12; Parry and Parry, *The Rise of the Medical Profession*, p. 105.
27. Jacyna, *Philosophic Whigs*, p. 97; See also Haakonssen, *Medicine and Morals in the Enlightenment*, p. 15; Loudon, *Medical Care and the General Practitioner*, p. 195.
28. Loudon, *Medical Care and the General Practitioner*, p. 275.
29. Faubert, *Rhyming Reason*, pp. 171–2. In his *ODNB* article on Brown, Stewart-Robinson notes that while '[h]e aspired to be an Akenside; his friends found him an embarrassment' and 'Dr James Gregory, with whom he entered into medical practice in 1806, regarded his amalgam of verse with philosophy as badly conceived.' For further on Duncan's poetry, see Faubert, *Rhyming Reason*, pp. 101–4.
30. On Duncan and club culture, see Chalmers, 'Medical Clubs and Societies', in Chalmers (ed.), *Andrew Duncan Senior, Physician of the Enlightenment*, pp. 114–33.
31. Duncan, *An Account of the Life, Writings, and Character, of the late Dr. Alexander Monro Secondus*, pp. vii–viii.
32. Cockburn, *Memorials of his Time*, p. 284.
33. Brown et al. (eds), *The Edinburgh History of Scottish Literature. Volume Two*, p. 205, p. 211, p. 216.
34. 'Macnish's *An Introduction to Phrenology*', *PJ*, 10 (1836–7), 552–6 (p. 552).
35. Findlay, *Robert Burns and the Medical Profession*, p. 97.
36. Thomas Aird, 'Memoir', in *The Poetical Works of David Macbeth Moir*, ed. by Thomas Aird, 2 vols (Edinburgh and London: William Blackwood and Sons, 1852), vol. 1, pp. xv–cxxxii (p. xxiv).
37. D. M. Moir to William Blackwood, 30 July 1820, NLS MS 4005, fols 236–7.
38. D. M. Moir to William Blackwood, 7 August 1820, NLS MS 4005, fols 238–9.
39. Clarke, *Autobiographical Recollections of the Medical Profession*, p. 489.

40. Blackwood refers to Moir by name in a letter dated 19 October 1820, NLS MS 30304, fols 168–9.

41. [D. M. Moir], 'Why are Professional Men Indifferent Poets?', *BEM*, 8 (January 1821), 415–19 (pp. 416, 418).

42. [J. G. Lockhart], 'On the Cockney School of Poetry. No. IV', *BEM*, 3 (August 1818), 519–24 (p. 519).

43. Ibid. p. 522, p. 524.

44. On the political motivations of this critique, see Roe, *John Keats and the Culture of Dissent*, pp. 160–81.

45. As Nicolas Roe notes, Maginn referred to Keats as 'the pharmacopolitical poet of Endymion' in a letter to Blackwood of 10 April 1821 (Roe, *John Keats and the Culture of Dissent*, p. 162); [Moir], 'Why are Professional Men Indifferent Poets?', p. 418.

46. [Moir], 'Why are Professional Men Indifferent Poets?', p. 415.

47. For an example from Moir's poetry, see *The Poetical Works of David Macbeth Moir*, vol. 1, p. 218.

48. [J. G. Lockhart], 'Remarks on Schlegel's History of Literature', *BEM*, 3 (August 1818), 497–510 (p. 498).

49. [Moir], 'Why are Professional Men Indifferent Poets?', p. 419.

50. [D. M. Moir], 'On Castle-Building', *Edinburgh Magazine and Literary Miscellany*, 10 (January 1822), 40–3 (p. 42).

51. [D. M. Moir], 'On Vulgar Prejudices Against Literature', *BEM*, 9 (May 1821), 173–9 (p. 176).

52. Roberts and Porter, 'Introduction', in Roberts and Porter (eds), *Literature & Medicine during the Eighteenth Century*, pp. 1–2.

53. Seward, *Anna Seward's Life of Erasmus Darwin*, p. 58.

54. Higgins, *Romantic Genius and the Literary Magazine*, p. 28.

55. [Moir], 'On Vulgar Prejudices Against Literature', p. 176, p. 177.

56. Ibid. p. 176.

57. Ibid. p. 178. For further on *Blackwood's* and Schlegel, see Duncan, '*Blackwood's* and Romantic Nationalism'.

58. [Moir], 'On Vulgar Prejudices Against Literature', p. 178.

59. Duncan, '*Blackwood's* and Romantic Nationalism', p. 76.

60. [Wilson], 'Noctes Ambrosianæ. No. LI', p. 418.

61. D. M. Moir to William Blackwood, 2 January 1830 [corrected as 1831], NLS MS 4030, fols 189–90.

62. On Galt and conjectural history, see Hewitt, 'Introduction: Observations and Conjectures on John Galt's Place in Scottish Enlightenment and Romantic-era Studies'.

63. John Galt to D. M. Moir, 4 September 1830, NLS Acc. 9856, No. 42.

64. John Galt to D. M. Moir, 21 September 1830, NLS Acc. 9856, No. 42.

65. D. M. Moir to William Blackwood, postmarked 31 January 1831, NLS MS 4030, fols 193–4.

66. D. M. Moir to William Blackwood, [1831?], NLS MS 4030, fols 219–20.

67. D. M. Moir to William Blackwood, postmarked 31 January 1831, NLS MS 4030, fols 193–4.

68. Allard, 'Medicine', p. 380.

69. Huisman and Warner, 'Medical Histories', p. 5, p. 6. See also Risse, 'Historicism in Medical History'.

70. Allard, 'Medicine', p. 380.

71. Barfoot, 'Philosophy and Method in Cullen's Medical Teaching', p. 118.

72. Ibid. p. 119. Barfoot is quoting from *The works of William Cullen, M.D. . . . containing his physiology, nosology, and first lines of the practice of physic: with numerous extracts from his manuscript papers, and from his treatise of the materia medica.* Ed. Thomson, J., 2 vols (Edinburgh: Blackwood, 1827), vol. 1, p. 375. For further on Cullen and also John Thomson on philosophy, see Shuttleton, '*An Account of . . . William Cullen:* John Thomson and the Making of a Medical Biography', in Coyer and Shuttleton (eds), *Scottish Medicine and Literary Culture*, pp. 240–66.

73. Moir, *Outlines of the Ancient History of Medicine*, p. 92.

74. Ibid. p. 94.

75. [D. M. Moir], 'Wonderful Passage in the Life of Mansie Wauch, Tailor', *BEM*, 16 (October 1824), 456–9 (p. 457, p. 456).

76. Ibid. p. 456.

77. [D. M. Moir], 'From the Autobiography of Mansie Wauch. Benjie on the Carpet,' *BEM*, 21 (January 1827), 39–44 (p. 41).

78. Ibid. p. 41.

79. Marshall, *Murdering to Dissect*. For further, see Richardson, *Death, Dissection and the Destitute*, p. 144.

80. Rosner, *The Anatomy Murders*, pp. 256–7.

81. [Robert Gooch], 'A Bill for Preventing the Unlawful Disinterment of Human Bodies, and for Regulating Schools of Anatomy', *QR*, 42 (January 1830), 1–17 (p. 17).

82. For an overview, see Haakonssen, *Medicine and Morals in the Enlightenment*, pp. 1–45, and in particular, p. 27; Guerrini, 'Alexander Monro *Primus* and the Moral Theatre of Anatomy'.

83. Aird, 'Memoir', p. xli.

84. Abercrombie, *Inquiries Concerning the Intellectual Powers and the Investigation of Truth*, p. 435.

85. Ibid. p. 433.

86. Ibid. p. 429.

87. Ibid. p. 177.

88. Ibid. p. 177.

89. Ibid. p. 180, p. 181.

90. Ibid. pp. 429–30.

91. Moir, *The Modern Pythagorean*, vol. 1, pp. 91–2.

92. See Barfoot, 'Philosophy and Method in Cullen's Medical Teaching', pp. 110–32.

93. 'Inquiries concerning the Intellectual Powers, and the investigation of Truth. By John Abercrombie, M.D.', *EMSJ*, 35 (1831), 401–26 (p. 401).

94. '*Outlines of the Ancient History of Medicine; being a View of the Healing Art among the Egyptians, Greeks, Romans, and Arabians*. By D. M. Moir', *Edinburgh Literary Journal*, No. 131 (14 May 1831), p. 307.

95. Moir, *Outlines of the Ancient History of Medicine*, p. 40.

96. Ibid. p. 40.

97. D. M. Moir to William Blackwood, postmarked 31 January 1831, NLS MS 4030, fols 193–4.

98. Macnish, as quoted in Moir, *The Modern Pythagorean*, vol. 1, p. 219.

99. William Blackwood to D. M. Moir, [no date], NLS Acc. 9856, No. 38.

100. D. M. Moir to [William Blackwood], 24 January 1830, NLS MS 4028, fols 54–55.

101. [D. M. Moir], 'On Medical Literature and Education', *Edinburgh Literary Gazette*, 2 (20 January 1830), 65–7 (p. 65).

102. On this wider deprecation, see Fisher, '"In the Present Famine of Anything Substantial"', p. 108.

103. [D. M. Moir], 'Letters to the Learned Professions. No. I. To the Students of Medicine', *FM*, 5 (March 1832), 238–43 (p. 238). On *Fraser's* and quackery, see below, p. 154.

104. 'Manual of the Economy of the Human Body', *Edinburgh Literary Gazette*, 2 (16 January 1830), 37–8 (p. 37).

105. [Moir], 'Letters to the Learned Professions', p. 241.

106. Ibid. p. 242.

107. Ibid. p. 242.

108. Moir, *Outlines of the Ancient History of Medicine*, p. iv.

109. 'To the Editor of the London Medical Gazette', *LMG*, 5 (14 November 1829), 209–10 (p. 209).

110. 'Dr Moir's Outlines of the Ancient History of Medicine', *LMG*, 8 (18 June 1831), 368–72 (p. 368).

111. [Moir], 'Letters to the Learned Professions', p. 239.

112. Rosner, *Medical Education in the Age of Improvement*, p. 176.
113. Ibid. p. 177.
114. Ibid. p. 191, p. 190.
115. John Abercrombie to Professor Russell as quoted in [Thomson], *Observations on the Preparatory Education of Candidates for the Degree of Doctor of Medicine*, pp. 7–8.
116. See [Thomson], *Hints Respecting the Improvement of the Literary & Scientific Education of Candidates for the Degree of Doctor of Medicine in the University of Edinburgh*, p. 9; [Moir], 'Letters to the Learned Professions', p. 239.
117. [Moir], 'Letters to the Learned Professions', p. 240.
118. Ibid. p. 241.
119. Richardson, *Death, Dissection and the Destitute*, p. 93.
120. [D. M. Moir], 'The Wounded Spirit', *FM*, 1 (May 1830), 417–26 (p. 425).
121. [D. M. Moir], 'The Wounded Spirit', *FM*, 1 (July 1830), 663–72 (p. 663, p. 664).
122. Abercrombie, *Inquiries Concerning the Intellectual Powers*, p. 435.
123. Haakonssen, *Medicine and Morals in the Enlightenment*, p. 27. See also Wayne Wild, 'The Origins of a Modern Medical Ethics in Enlightenment Scotland', in Coyer and Shuttleton (eds), *Scottish Medicine and Literary Culture*, pp. 48–73.
124. Ibid. p. 27; for further on Gregory and religion, see Passmore, *Fellows of Edinburgh's College of Physicians*, p. 57.
125. Aird, 'Memoir', p. lxvi.
126. [D. M. Moir], 'Sabbath. In Six Sonnets. By Delta', *BEM*, 22 (November 1827), 610–11 (p. 610).
127. W. Lindsay Alexander, 'Delta and his Writings', *Hogg's Weekly Instructor*, 4 (1855), 173–82 (p. 181).
128. Ibid. p. 173.
129. Ibid. p. 173.
130. 'David Macbeth Moir, (Delta)', *MacPhail's Edinburgh Ecclesiastical Journal*, 80 (September 1852), 65–76 (p. 68); 'Poetical Resemblances', *Hogg's Weekly Instructor*, 1 (3 May 1845), 145–6 (p. 146).
131. Aird, 'Memoir', p. lxiv.
132. Ibid. pp. lxiv–lxv.
133. [Moir], *Domestic Verses*, p. 8.
134. Ibid. p. 12, p. 18.
135. Aird, 'Memoir', p. cxxxii.
136. 'David Macnish Moir, (Delta)', pp. 72–3.
137. Examples include: D. M. Moir's letters to William Blackwood: 22 February [1821], NLS MS 4007, fols 152–3; 7 December 1826, NLS

MS 4018, fols 57–8; [1828?], NLS MS 4022, fols 174–5; 22 February 1830, NLS MS 4028, fols 58–9; 5 March 1830, NLS MS 4028, fols 60–1; 26 November 1832, NLS MS 4034, fols 76–7; [1832?], NLS MS 4034, fols 84–5.

138. Aird, 'Memoir', p. xl.
139. [W. E. Aytoun], 'The Late D. M. Moir,' *BEM*, 70 (August 1851), 249–50 (p. 250).
140. On Moir and cholera, see Pitman, 'David M. Moir: Cholera Papers'.
141. Richardson, *Death, Dissection and the Destitute*, p. 223, p. 227, p. 226.
142. As quoted in Moir, *The Modern Pythagorean*, vol. 1, p. 213.
143. Ibid. pp. 210–22. As Pitman's reading of Moir's cholera papers held at the Royal College of Physicians of Edinburgh reveals, Moir also corresponded with individual laypersons regarding the efficacy of various treatment options (Pitman, 'David M. Moir: Cholera Papers', pp. 545–6).
144. In March 1832, Moir writes to Blackwood relating how his contribution to the contagionist debate has already forwarded his medical reputation (D. M. Moir to William Blackwood, 25 March 1832, NLS MS 4034, fols 65–6).
145. [Aytoun], 'The Late D. M. Moir', p. 250.
146. [D. M. Moir], 'Echoes of Antiquity. – By Delta. I. – Hippocrates to the Ambassadors of Artaxerxes', *BEM*, 40 (December 1836), 781–3 (p. 781, p. 782).
147. Ibid. p. 783; Moir, *The Modern Pythagorean*, vol. 1, p. 123.
148. For example, see 'The Poetical Works of David Macbeth Moir', *The Literary Gazette* (1 May 1852), 381–2; 'The Poetry of David Moir', *Sharpe's London Magazine* (1 July 1852), 56–9; 'David Macbeth Moir', *Tait's Edinburgh Magazine* (19 June 1852), 327–30.
149. 'The Poetical Works of David Macbeth Moir ("Delta")', *The New Quarterly Review and Digest of Current Literature*, 1 (July 1852), 30–1 (p. 30).
150. 'David Macbeth Moir', p. 327.
151. On religious biography in the periodical press, Topham, 'The *Wesleyan-Methodist Magazine* and religious monthlies in early nineteenth-century Britain', in Cantor et al. (eds), *Science in the Nineteenth-Century Periodical*, pp. 67–90.
152. *Sketches of Eminent Medical Men*, pp. 5–6.
153. Christie, '*Blackwood's Edinburgh Magazine* in the Scientific Culture of Early Nineteenth-Century Edinburgh', in Morrison and Roberts (eds), *Romanticism and Blackwood's Magazine*, 125–36.

154. Warren, 'Preface to the Present Edition', in *Passages from the Diary of a Late Physician*, People's Edition, p. vi.
155. Porter, *Bodies Politic*, p. 258. See also Loudon, *Medical Care and the General Practitioner*, pp. 267–96.
156. Sparks, *The Doctor in the Victorian Novel*, p. 14.
157. Ibid. p. 13.
158. See Rothfield, 'Medicine'. For further on Brown, see Coyer, 'The Medical Kailyard'. On Maclaren, see below, pp. 210–12.
159. Aird, 'Memoir', p. cxxx, p. cxx.

Chapter 4

Professionalisation and the Case of Samuel Warren's *Passages from the Diary of a Late Physician*

From the publication of the first chapter in *Blackwood's* in August 1830 to the appearance of a 'People's Edition' in 1854, Warren's *Passages from the Diary of a Late Physician* was an international literary sensation. Written from the perspective of a late physician who recounts the 'secret history' of the medical profession, including his own 'Early Struggles' to become a prominent physician in London, the series consisted of sketches of notable medical cases, which range from the macabre to the sentimental.[1] The first separately published volumes appeared in America, under the title *Affecting Scenes; Being Passages from the Diary of a Physician* (1831), prior to the publication of the first Edinburgh edition in 1832. It went through at least seven editions in Britain prior to the publication of the People's Edition, and was translated into French and German. According to Warren's letters to Blackwood, one chapter was even 'translated in to the native Cherokee language!!!'[2]

This period of immense popular currency coincides with the key decades for the professionalisation of medicine in Britain. Between 1830 and 1858, 'medical knowledge became more scientific, medical education more systematic, and the medical profession more unified'.[3] Prior to the Medical Act of 1858, elite medical corporations, the highest ranking of which was the Royal College of Physicians of London, controlled the licensing of practitioners, but the act created the General Medical Council and made registration with the GMC the new benchmark for professionalism.[4] As Magali Sarfatti Larson notes, this represented 'a victory of the middle class against aristocratic privilege'.[5] Specialist scientific knowledge, gained through a systematic medical education and evidenced by registration with the GMC, became the mark of the 'regular' practitioner (finally distinguishing him from the 'fringe' or 'quack' practitioners with whom he competed in the medical marketplace), and the traditional tripartite hierarchy between physicians, surgeons, and apothecaries became increasingly irrelevant.[6] However, while the Medical Act of 1858 represents a key legislative shift, such changes occurred gradually throughout the period, and the garnering of social esteem for the profession, particularly from the growing middle-class medical consumer market, was vital to this process. For example, as S. E. D. Shortt explains, the rhetorical display of scientific knowledge was far more important in forwarding professional authority than the actual science itself.[7] There was perhaps no better medium to reach this audience and to perform such rhetorical displays than the popular periodical press.

Warren's series has been read as both contributing to and detracting from the agenda of professionalisation. Heather Worthington builds upon the work of Peter Drexler, reading Warren's series as contributing to a popular genre of professional anecdotes becoming increasingly pervasive through the middle of the nineteenth century, which 'served both to consolidate and to popularise the status of the emergent professional classes'.[8] Her focus is upon how Warren's *Diary* 'inaugurate[s] the case structure that will typify later detective fiction, and, in the figure of the observing and analytic physician, explore a discursive space that will later be occupied by the disciplinary detective in the private sphere'.[9] However, her reading of the late physician as an exemplification of growing disciplinary power stands in stark contrast to Meegan Kennedy's assertion that,

> although Warren's case histories strove to enlist the reader's benevolent identification with a physician portrayed as hardworking and sensitive, the narrator's exaggerated sympathy, overbearing moralization, and curious interests ultimately represented a challenge to the nineteenth-century medical community, which aimed to produce itself as objective, professional, discreet, and above all truthful.[10]

The key difference in their interpretations hinges upon Kennedy's account of the case history as a genre that highlights the rhetorical policing of nineteenth-century medicine – as a key site for the (at least attempted) excision of the 'curious' discourses of eighteenth-century medicine and for the portrayal of nineteenth-century medicine as objective and scientific. The late physician as a medical 'man of feeling', deeply interested in his patients' lives, whose cases appeal to the same voyeuristic desires as the earlier Blackwoodian tales of terror, may have threatened such a representation. However, the late physician, like the 'gentle' surgeon and poet Delta, may also be read as an ideal moral and religious medico-literary figure – as part of the 'neo-Mackenzian revival of "feeling"' in Romantic-era Edinburgh – and as participating in a much wider public relations campaign that was also vital to the development of medical authority in the nineteenth century.[11]

This chapter reads the series in its vexed original publishing context – the ideologically charged popular periodical press – in terms of its inception and reception, as well as its initiation of a new genre of medico-popular writing, and places this reading in relation to debates surrounding the professionalisation of medicine, which included not only the importance of scientific practices but also a humanistic, and often Christian, outlook. In this I argue that Warren's series follows in the tradition of medical ethics initiated by John Gregory. With its avowed mission to reunite intellect and feeling in all arenas of social and intellectual life, *Blackwood's* provided an ideal platform for the construction of a professional medical man of feeling – even though the series was originally intended for one of its major competitors, Henry Colburn's *New Monthly Magazine*.

The *New Monthly Magazine* and the False Start of the Late Physician

Henry Colburn founded the *New Monthly Magazine* in 1814 to counter the Jacobin tendencies of the *Monthly Magazine* and to capitalise on the surge of anti-Jacobin feeling following the defeat of Napoleon at Waterloo.[12] However, in contrast to *Blackwood's*, the ideology of the *New Monthly* was rooted more firmly in liberal economics than in party politics, and when the Tory-leaning Colburn relaunched the magazine in 1821, with the Whig poet Thomas Campbell as editor, he intended to meet the demands of a middle-class audience, avowedly separating literature and politics, emphasising original literature, and thus providing 'a pleasant diversion from the care of middle-class life'.[13] While Campbell was known to be politically uncontroversial and happy to provide a 'calm spot' amid the politicised periodical press, his sub-editor, Cyrus Redding, was a more outspoken supporter of reform.[14] The result, as Nanora Sweet explains, was not an entirely apolitical magazine, but rather a 'dialectical product (Tory, Whig, Radical) of its three individual coadjutors', well-adapted 'to the liberal coalition-building that replaced strict partisanship in the 1820s'.[15]

Campbell, Redding, and Colburn themselves maintained a successful coalition until September 1830, when Redding resigned, disgruntled with Colburn's management of the magazine. According to Redding's *Fifty Years' Recollections, Literary and Personal* (1858), it was the handling of Warren's *Diary* that led to the final break. Redding relates that Warren sent him the first chapter in 1829, and seeing its 'merits', he 'sent it off to the printer, sealed and directed as usual'.[16] However, some of Colburn's employees interfered with his judgement, representing the chapter as unfit for publication, and Colburn, without Redding's knowledge, rejected what would become one of the most popular periodical publications of its day.

In the editorial introduction to 'Early Struggles', evidently written after the work was accepted for *Blackwood's*, Warren celebrates the Blackwoodian context. Appropriately, his 'series of extracts from a late physician's diary' will appear 'in a Magazine, which was the first to present papers of this class to the public'.[17] In this statement he is not implying that *Blackwood's* regularly published physicians' diaries. Rather, the magazine was known for presenting supposedly 'original' documents and accounts to the 'prying gaze of the public'.[18] (Maga was, of course, also known for her hoaxes.) Instead, 'one solitary paper, which appeared in a contemporaneous Magazine* some months ago, and which professed to be the first of a series' is identified as the only real precursor to his work. An editorial note informs the reader that the 'contemporaneous Magazine' to which the editor refers is the *New Monthly*.[19]

Despite his emphasis on the precursor being 'one solitary paper', Warren is almost certainly referring to a series of three articles entitled 'The Young Surgeon', published in the *New Monthly* between April and July 1829, which consisted of a young surgeon's first-hand account of his medical education, famous teachers and associates in

London and Edinburgh, and some early cases. The *Wellesley Index of Victorian Periodicals* attributes 'The Young Surgeon' as most probably written by Warren himself and interprets his reference to the *New Monthly* as a deliberate 'puff' of his own previous work. Reading the *Diary*, and 'Early Struggles' in particular, as a continuation of a discursive strand regarding contemporary medical practice begun in the *New Monthly*, sheds a distinct ideological light on the beginnings of Warren's series. As we will see, in the Blackwoodian context the series is best viewed as a new development of the tale of terror, in which the genre re-coalesces with the case history, a continuation of the morally didactic and implicitly conservative mode of Wilson's proto-Kailyard writings, and a seminal and highly controversial depiction of North's ideal literary and gentlemanly medical man. However, in the context of the *New Monthly*, intra-professional politics and issues surrounding medical reform instead come to the fore.

From its inception, the *New Monthly* contained a remarkable number of original papers devoted exclusively to medical topics. As such, Warren's inclination to publish in its pages is unsurprising. A survey of the magazine from 1814 through 1829 reveals four series of original papers devoted to medicine, as well as a series of medical extracts (often from medical journals or larger works) entitled 'Medical Miscellanies'. The first of the original medical series, 'The Guardian of Health', which ran from March 1814 through May 1816, presented practical medical information to a popular audience and was intended to enable readers 'not only to dispense on a hundred occasions with the aid of the physician, but likewise to distinguish the man of real skill from the mere pretender'.[20] The first number is 'On the Character of Physicians' and delineates the qualities of a true physician as 'a due share of learning, a sound understanding, and a noble and feeling heart'.[21] This fusion of popular advice and reverence for the 'regular' medical professional is continued in 'The Physician', which ran from September 1822 through November 1824, and claimed to be 'from the pen of an eminent Physician'.[22]

Following the conclusion of this series, the medical papers of the *New Monthly* shifted towards a focus on the individual medical professional, rather than the provision of advice – a shift commercially in tune with the growing interest in medical biography. The surgeon Thomas Richards (1800–77) contributed a series of 'Professional

Sketches' between November 1828 and April 1829, which not only celebrated eminent medical and surgical men but also lauded them as middle-class heroes who had improved medical science and gained status through merit and hard work, while their lesser contemporaries merely lined their pockets by appealing to an embarrassingly outmoded patronage system.[23] John Abernethy, for example, is celebrated for his lack of polish, distinguished by his dedication to scientific practice over regard for professional status from that 'cringing pulse-feeling race'.[24]

The *New Monthly* was a magazine designed to appeal to the rising professional middle classes, and Mark Parker defines its overarching ideology to be one of 'liberal bourgeois capitalism'. According to Parker, through the 1820s it consistently 'attacks the idle ceremonial aristocracy, champions free trade, worries about popular unrest, advocates freedom of the press and the free exchange of ideas, and asserts selection by merit over connection or caste'.[25] The magazine's fascination with the medical profession, and in particular its sympathies towards medical reform, are therefore unsurprising. The most explicit example is perhaps the third number of Richards' 'Professional Sketches', devoted to 'Dr. Armstrong and the College of Physicians' and published in January 1829. The sketch is primarily a vehement critique of the RCP of London and its sole concern with protecting its own rights and privileges and maintaining 'that imposing dignity, with which its own members only have invested it'.[26] Rather than policing malpractice amongst licensed medical practitioners or working to minimise the activities of unqualified quack practitioners, according to Richards, the RCP instead focuses its attention on harassing respectable and well-educated medical practitioners such as Dr Edward Harrison, who dared to write prescriptions in London without RCP licensure. John Armstrong (1784–1829) is said to have been treated in the 'same aristocratic style as Dr Harrison; his admission as a Licentiate being opposed in a manner, and with a degree of acrimony, that will reflect no credit upon the "august" tribunal, whose business it is to regulate these matters'.[27] He is presented as one who, while attempting to establish himself in London with 'scanty' advantages, dares 'to dissent from the majority of his elders' in working to improve the understanding and treatment of typhus fever.[28] Reform, motivated by the 'nobler principle' of 'doing good', is juxtaposed against the aristocratic practices of the RCP.[29]

Further, in praising Armstrong for his liberality and kindness 'in his conduct toward the younger members of the profession', Richards emphasises the rarity of such conduct, particularly amongst the senior Fellows of the RCP, whose requisite 'gentlemanly' Oxbridge degrees are clearly no guard against 'downright rudeness'.[30]

The *London Medical Gazette* came to the RCP's rescue by printing a rebuttal to Richards' series as a lead article the following month. The article on 'Professional Puffs' decries his 'Sketches' as not only inaccurate but also hurtful to the medical men featured, who are degraded as the subjects of vulgar puffing.[31] In turn, the polemical leader of the medical reform movement, *The Lancet*, printed a response from 'The Author of the "Professional Sketches"', which emphatically reaffirms the 'dirty behaviour' of the Fellows towards younger members of the profession.[32] This 'dirty behaviour', as detailed in the 'Sketches', includes the purposeful undermining of young practitioners' access to lucrative patients, foreshadowing the late physician's experience in 'Early Struggles'.

'Early Struggles' re-enacts what Dorothy and Roy Porter have identified as a prevalent myth of the 'great doctor' who establishes himself through a chance encounter with a wealthy patron who then enables him to lay the foundation for a fashionable practice.[33] Prior to this providential encounter, the late physician is almost entirely without patients, and he and his dutiful young wife face the same miseries of deprivation, and resultant ill health, that he will later attempt to alleviate for others. Had Redding's acceptance of Warren's manuscript not been blocked, its depiction of the haughty and dismissive character of the established practitioners whom the late physician encounters during his 'Early Struggles' would have furthered the *New Monthly*'s critique of the medical aristocracy.

When the late physician first gains admittance into a fashionable house to treat a wealthy gentleman for an asthmatic affliction, the family physician, Sir—, is displeased with his presence and sends the patient, Sir William, away to Worthing for a change of air. This both disables the late physician from treating Sir William and also quickly leads to the patient's death. The late physician laments: 'There is nothing in the world so easy, as for the eminent members of our profession to take the bread out of the mouths of their younger brethren, with the best grace in the world.'[34] At this point he has already suffered at the hands of a 'late celebrated' physician, who made him appear unknowledgeable in front of a patient and thus rendered his future services undesirable,[35] and he soon resorts to applying to 'a very celebrated and successful brother practitioner' for temporary financial relief. He imagines the reception his note might meet: 'I tried to put myself in the place of him I had written to, and fancy the feelings with which I should receive a similar application.'[36] However, the feelings of the 'brother practitioner' are not in his favour. He sends the trifle of a guinea and writes in return 'that when young men attempt a station in life without competent funds to meet it, they cannot wonder if they fail'.[37] For the late physician, 'recollections of past times' serve to moderate his feelings when he himself achieves eminence, as he determines never to turn a 'deaf ear to applications from the younger and less successful members' of the profession.[38]

Despite the late physician's seemingly admirable behaviour towards his younger brethren, the context of the series in the *New Monthly* would have prompted readers to view his character satirically rather than sympathetically. If Warren was also the author of 'The Young Surgeon', which followed immediately on from the final number of Richards' 'Sketches' in April 1829, he developed a strikingly different voice for the late physician – one with far greater melodramatic flair. The late physician's criticisms of the medical elite appear somewhat ludicrous in light of his own indignant pride in his Cambridge degree and his resultant standing as a gentleman and a scholar. When forced to give classics lessons to avoid starvation, he declares, 'a gentleman, and a member of an English University, was driven so low as to attend, for these terms, an ignorant underling', and he is deeply insulted when called in to treat 'servants, housekeepers, porters' and, most tryingly of all, the 'favourite pointer' of an 'insulting coxcomb'.[39] Eventually, he decries his own 'egregious vanity', which has prevented him from accepting the perhaps more lucrative but 'humbler sphere of the general practitioner', even though his single interaction with a general practitioner (who incidentally refuses to hire him) is marked by feelings of repulsion towards this 'vulgar fellow'.[40] Richards' 'Sketches' had defended the worth of the general practitioner against such dismissive elitism just a few months prior, and the late physician's egoistical complaint stands in stark contrast to the staid and reflective voice of 'The Young Surgeon', who despite being the son of a 'gentleman' is in training for the humbler lot of the surgeon.[41] Further, while

the surgeon's praise for the medical education available at Edin-
burgh and the newly founded London University accords with the
New Monthly's favourable account of the 'Progress of the London
University' in April 1829, the late physician's high valuation of his
Cambridge degree and gentlemanly status would have sat uneasily
in the magazine.[42]

If 'Early Struggles' may have been read satirically in the *New
Monthly*, in the pages of *Blackwood's* the late physician becomes a
realisation of the ideal moral and religious medical practitioner –'your
man of education – your scholar and your gentleman'.[43] Beyond the
endorsement of extra-professional literary pursuits in the *Noctes
Ambrosianæ*, discussed in Chapter 3, North praises the gentlemanly
character of Dr Clark and the popular nature of his treatise on climate
in the number that introduces Warren's series, expressing his 'hope
that other physicians will lay aside the stilts and the veil'.[44] Such a
framing context appears to have been carefully calculated to produce
a sympathetic reception for the late physician's literary unmasking of
the 'secret history' of the medical profession.[45] *Blackwood's* also, of
course, had little grief with Oxbridge.

A Blackwoodian Hoax

The reputation of medical men was at a low ebb following the anatomy murders, and while Warren himself was not a medical man,
the *Diary* became an extended, if often contested, public relations
campaign, galvanised by a prototypically Blackwoodian hoax.
Warren was a lawyer by trade, but his series was presented to the
public as a genuine 'diary' of a late physician until the Edinburgh
edition of 1838, in which he publicly avowed his authorship. As he
explains in the 1838 edition, he 'engaged in the practical study of
physic' prior to beginning his legal career,[46] but in an apparent deviation from his original career plans, in 1828 he was admitted into
the Inner Temple, London to study law and in 1831 commenced
practice as a special pleader, calling at the bar in 1837 and becoming
Queen's Counsel in 1851.[47] Despite his eventual success, Warren's
early letters to William Blackwood contain evidence of his own early
struggles and refer to an expensive chancery suit that plagued him
during his legal studies. In a later letter to Alexander Blackwood, he

reflects that 'the "Diary" was begun by me to ~~xxx~~ save myself from literal starvation'.[48] We might surmise then that his hoax on the reading public was, at least in part, a device designed to guarantee the popularity, and hence the lucrativeness, of the series.

Warren at first kept his identity secret from even Blackwood himself, but after he revealed his identity to Blackwood in December 1830 the publisher congratulated him on his 'incognito', declaring that 'the very mystery and conjecture as to the author of a series of popular papers add to their interest'.[49] Revelling in the public's fascination with the authorship of the papers and their various speculations regarding which great medical man must be responsible, Blackwood writes to Warren in February 1831:

> An uncommonly clever lady, Mrs Dr Hughes, an old friend of mine, wrote me the other day that there was a very general idea in London that the late Dr Gooch's papers had afforded the materials for these interesting Papers. I am quite amused at the speculation which the strict incognito causes. Let the good folks wonder on.[50]

Moir and Macnish, who, like Gooch, were known to contribute to *Blackwood's*, along with eminent physicians such as Matthew Baillie (1761–1823), the same John Armstrong harassed by the RCP (not the medical poet), and John Ayrton Paris (*bap.* 1785–*d.* 1856), were all discussed as possible candidates by the reading public.[51] Warren was annoyed when the Paris edition was published under the name of William Harrison (1812–60), who was not a medical man but had 'written a long since dead-and-damned book called "Tales of a Physician"'.[52] Warren may not have been the very first to write in this genre, but he was proud of being the first to do it well.

While gaining popularity through curious intrigue and thus ensuring Blackwood's continued interest in publishing further chapters, the hoax also brought the series to the attention of the medical profession. Perhaps most strikingly, in August 1830, a correspondent writing 'To the Editor of The Lancet' on 'Blackwood's Magazine, v. the Secrets of the Medical Profession', claims that though the *Diary* bears the 'indubitable marks of *fiction*', he fears that the disclosure of '*the sacred secrets which are communicated to us in perfect confidence by our patients*' to the general public might lead to the distrust of physicians.[53] Responding to *The Lancet's* critique in a

'Note to the Editor' in *Blackwood's* in October 1830, Warren points out that medical journals routinely publish narrative case histories with a similar level of detail and are often found in the hands of the interested lay person.[54] The *London Medical Gazette* was more staid, defending the author of the series against any supposed breach of patient confidence, but only on the grounds that it was so evidently a ruse.[55]

In response to such critiques, Warren was keen to ensure that Blackwood was aware that both the medical profession and the reading public were not unanimously against nor entirely unconvinced by his series. In a letter of September 1830, he notes that he has shown his latest chapter, 'Intriguing and Madness', to a medical man in London who praised its accurate depiction of 'a strong mind's madness'.[56] The following month, he notes complacently that 'Dr Birkbeck (he of Mechanic Institutes celebrity)' is 'wild' about his series:

> He is making every exertion to discover who is the writer of them; and he, and a man of some station, had actually (so they told a friend of mine) searched among upwards of 40 physicians living and dead – but in vain. At this moment there is lying on my desk a very flattering note written by Dr. B— to a gay friend of mine – begging him to forward me a ticket to a public place 'with his compliments' &c!![57]

Warren also had a habit of 'accidentally' being discovered as the author of the series by his own medical consultants. He claims that when 'one of the most eminent Hospital-Surgeons in London' came to his house, he happened to see a draft lying on his desk and declared, '"I hear of them among my patients every where I go."' According to Warren, he concludes: '"'tis a thousand pities you are not in our profession" – said he "what a <u>business</u> your papers would have brought you!"' Warren takes advantage of this encounter to ask whether 'any parts are over-charged – exaggerated', and the answer is, unsurprisingly, reported to be that the late physician's descriptions are utterly accurate. Warren also takes advice on 'the professional <u>accuracy of detail</u> concerning the disease in the spine' in 'The Martyr-Philosopher' and notes that the surgeon has supplied him with 'some prodigiously interesting materials for future chapters – or perhaps, towards some future <u>series</u> of chapters'.[58] According to Warren's letters to Blackwood, another medical consultant, when treating him for cholera in 1832, refuses to take a fee from him as he 'considered it an honour to attend me who by his writings had done more to elevate the medical profession in public estimation, than had been done for the last 50 years'.[59]

Moir and Macnish, genuine medical contributors to *Blackwood's*, were rather less enthusiastic about the series. Writing to Moir in October 1831, Macnish asks:

> Have you ever heard the name of the writer of the Physician's Diary? I have more than once heard it attributed to yourself. It has been exceedingly popular, though I confess I do not like it so well as most people. I question much indeed if it be written by a medical man at all. I suppose it is the handywork of some gemman of the press in London who has picked up a few medical phrases.[60]

Moir was similarly suspicious. In September 1830 he writes to Blackwood that '[a] medical man's they can scarcely be, as many of the details are quite out of keeping both with a Doctor's feelings and experiences'. However, ever attuned to assuring the magazine's success, he advises: 'The series seems to be much and generally liked _ Therefore by all manner of means encourage the writer to proceed with it.'[61] His primary critique of the series was that some chapters, such as 'Consumption', were 'very much overdrawn' and thus 'as the report of a <u>medical</u> person totally ridiculous'.[62] Regardless of his mixed feelings towards the *Diary*, however, the reading public was not entirely off base in suspecting that Delta might be the author of the controversial series. The critique of professional values put forth in Moir's earlier periodical writings is carried forward in the *Diary*, as the late physician becomes a hyperbolic model of the professional who still values 'generosity, romance, and chivalry' and sees in his patients '[m]an, "with the human face divine"'.[63]

The Medical Man of Feeling

The first chapter or 'case' to follow the late physician's account of his 'Early Struggles' establishes his character as a medical practitioner who, against criteria of medico-scientific professionalism based upon objectivity and the power of the medical gaze, values 'natural' affect as much as scientific practice. Simply entitled 'Cancer', the case describes an excruciating operation to remove a breast tumour. This takes place, of course, prior to the advent of anaesthesia, and the primary focus of the case is the young woman's extraordinary fortitude under a surgeon's knife. However, the physician's interactions with and reactions to the young wife and her plight provide the narrative frame, and the characterisation of the surgeon who performs the operation serves as an informative contrast, highlighting the uniqueness of the late physician. While the surgeon proceeds with preparations for the operation with 'a calm and business-like air', the late physician notes that upon seeing the surgical instruments laid out, 'I could scarce avoid a certain nervous tremor – unprofessional as it may seem.'[64] Many years of practice have yet to extinguish the physician's 'abhorrence, for the operative part of the profession', and the beauty of this particular patient appears to aggravate his emotional response.[65] The woman observes how '*very* kind and feeling' the late physician is towards her and asks him to hold a letter from her husband, who is away at sea, within her view, such that throughout the operation, she might steady herself by looking upon 'his dear handwriting'.[66] The physician sympathetically suffers with his patient throughout the surgery; ironically, the only thing that consoles him is his 'conviction of the consummate skill' of the surgeon, who 'with a calm eye, and a steady hand' flawlessly performs the operation.[67]

While the patient is the focus of the chapter, the late physician's humane character is a significant subtext. If, as Ruth Richardson has argued, 'by the turn of the nineteenth century, both the dead and the living body had alike become objectified, or "reified", within the anatomical and surgical fraternity', Warren's series re-humanises both the living body and the physician, while emphasising the paradoxical utility of objectification for the surgeon.[68] Perhaps Moir and Macnish's dislike of the series may in part be attributed to Warren's demarcation of the physician, in particular, as the gentlemanly, moral medical practitioner. Their own projected but never realised medico-literary collaboration was to be titled 'Lies, Pathetic and Humorous, by Moir, Macnish & Co. *Surgeons* and Tale Writers' (my italics), and in early 1831 Macnish attempted, unsuccessfully, to publish his own 'Passages in the Life of a Surgeon'.[69]

Like the Blackwoodian construction of Moir as an idealised medico-literary figure, the late physician's humanity is linked to his literary sensibilities. In the case entitled 'Consumption', published in November 1830, the delicate sensibility of the young, beautiful and tragically consumptive heiress is only rivalled by the physician's sympathetic sensibility towards her, which is enabled by his appreciation of her poetic and musical abilities – she is a lover of Dante, Milton, and Mozart. Beyond providing a clear example of the romanticisation of consumption famously discussed by Susan Sontag, the case emphasises the aesthetic foundations for the late physician's sympathy. In a melodramatic moment, when the young woman suddenly finds the strength to express herself through music one final time, the physician does 'not attempt to characterise the melting music which Miss B— was pouring from the piano' but rather reflects upon his own feelings:

> I have often thought that there is a sort of *spiritual*, unearthly character about some of the masses of Mozart, which draws out the greatest sympathies of one's nature, striking the deepest and most hidden chords of the human heart. On the present occasion, the peculiar circumstances in which I was placed – the time – the place – the dying angel whose hand was clasped in mind – disposed me to a more intense appreciation of Mozart's music than I had ever known before.[70]

The fine arts, as in Reid's account of the second class of natural signs, form the foundation of his understanding of the mind of the other. The patient's 'partiality for poetry' and her own poetic utterances, containing 'very beautiful thoughts, suggested by the bitterness of her own premature fate', likewise aid the development of the physician's intense sympathetic reaction.[71] If *Blackwood's* and Dr Peter Morris had declared that the study of literature, rather than philosophical introspection, was a better means to truly understand the 'most divine part of our nature', the late physician, following the prompt of Christopher North, applies this method to the study of his patients.[72]

Affecting Scenes and Tory Popular Literature

Meegan Kennedy's argument – that Warren's series threatened medico-scientific professionalism – depends upon her reading the text as a series of literary case histories, posing as real case histories, but deviating from the progressive rhetorical norms of clinical medicine (which included an attempted excision of any strong emotion). However, the case history is merely one of several traditions upon which Warren builds, and an important source for gauging the contemporary generic understanding of Warren's series – and thus the readerly expectations fostered by it – is the first separately published edition of the text, the *Affecting Scenes* of 1831.[73] Expanding upon Warren's original editorial introduction to 'Early Struggles', the 'Preface' to this edition reflects upon the moral salience of deathbed scenes and the particular interest of insights from those who stand upon that 'awful point, which separates time from eternity'.[74] Like Warren's introduction, the 'Preface' emphasises the medical man's privileged access to such scenes and the value of recording them intelligently for the benefit of wider society. The 'Preface' also expands upon the original text to highlight an important novelty of the *Diary*: its focus upon the deathbeds of ordinary persons. Noting the tendency of the age to publish accounts of the 'deathbed of some distinguished character', such as that of Joseph Addison, 'seen instructing a profligate [his stepson, the Earl of Warwick] how a Christian can meet death', the 'Preface' laments that 'those in humbler walks of life have been overlooked, as if men could be taught only by great examples'.[75]

The deathbed scene was a significant topos in eighteenth-century British literature, often exploited for its moralising potential. Besides the famous account of Addison's own virtuous death, he and Steele frequently included deathbed scenes in *The Spectator*, and Stephen Miller identifies Addison's tragedy *Cato* (1713), Samuel Richardson's novel *Clarissa* (1748), and Benjamin West's painting *The Death of General Wolfe* (1770) as '[t]he three most famous eighteenth-century English deathbed scenes'.[76] Within *Blackwood's*, De Quincey provides intimate details of Kant's deathbed in 'The Last Days of Immanuel Kant' (1827), while Sir Herbert Taylor's 'Memorandum' (1827) provides the 'most interesting and affecting Narrative' of the last illness and death of the Duke of York.[77] In shifting to humbler scenes, however, Warren was not entirely original. Moir, Galt, Hogg, Lockhart and Wilson, among others, populated the pages of *Blackwood's* with scenes from parochial Scottish life, and Wilson, in particular, had a penchant for the deathbed scene.

In 1831, when *Affecting Scenes* was published, Warren's series was still a work in progress, and the published tales would not quite fill two volumes. A 'Supplement' of five additional tales by other hands fills the second half of volume two. All but one of them, Galt's 'The Buried Alive', were taken from Wilson's *Lights and Shadows of Scottish Life* (1822), and all were first published in *Blackwood's* in the early 1820s. While Galt's medical tale of terror, with its horrific depiction of suspended animation and grave-robbing anatomists, has a clear continuity with tales from the *Diary*, such as 'Grave-Doings', in which the physician himself turns resurrectionist, and 'The Thunderstruck', which depicts a young girl's corpse-like catatonia, Wilson's tales have little medical content beyond a moralistic association of poor health with an uneasy mind. This association is likewise prevalent in the *Diary*, but Wilson's tales also complement Warren's in their focus on death and near-death experience and in their religious piety. In 'The Elder's Death-bed', for example, the narrator joins a minister who is on his way to the deathbed of a church elder, who not only dies an exemplary holy death, but also prompts a new faith in his disbelieving son, while 'The Elder's Funeral' (renamed 'The Penitent Son' in *Affecting Scenes*) depicts the elder's funeral in the rural kirkyard and confirms his son's repentance.

Wilson is traditionally considered one of the villains of Scottish literary history. Andrew Noble, for example, views Wilson's frequent literary deathbed scenes as 'the essential occasions for intensified guilt and hence repentance from sexual and radical sins' and accuses him of exploiting 'nationalism and religion in order to pursue class politics' to further the 'Tory hegemony'.[78] While *Lights and Shadows of Scottish Life* belongs to the early years of *Blackwood's*, in which the magazine emphasised the importance of imaginative literature as an 'index of national character and religious feeling', Wilson's text looks forward to what Philip Connell identifies as a post-1825 shift towards an increased attentiveness to a perceived need for a moral and religiously oriented 'paternalistic and dispensatory form of popular education'.[79] Medical subject matter was drawn upon in this particular strand of popular education, and Murray's 'Family Library' series, hailed by *Blackwood's* as the 'first *Tory* series of cheap books' designed to educate a mass public,[80] included the volume *Lives of British Physicians* (1830), in which the medical profession was celebrated for furnishing 'a larger proportion of names eminent for intellectual zeal and power, which have also deserved to be handed down for moral dignity of character, piety to God, and benevolence to man'.[81] Warren's series similarly utilised medical subject matter to advance the Tory cause, yoking the increased popular interest in 'medical lives' to extant models of Blackwoodian fiction.

From its offset, Warren presented his series as providing moral training for the reader, and this is made even more explicit in the preface to the People's Edition, where he writes of his desire to be viewed not as a 'Novelist', but as a 'MORALIST', and extracts Johnson's motto concerning fiction: 'These familiar histories may perhaps be made of greater use, than the solemnities of professed Morality; and convey the knowledge of Vice and Virtue with more efficacy, than axioms and definitions.'[82] 'A Scholar's Death-Bed' in September 1830, for example, is characteristically overt, opening with the hope 'that some young men of powerful, undisciplined, and ambitious minds, will find their account in an attentive consideration of the fate of a kindred spirit'.[83] The young, destitute scholar, an orphaned only son of humble parents, alone and dying of consumption, explains to the inquiring physician that he merits his current misery, exclaiming: 'I have indulged in wild ambitious hopes – lived in absurd dreams of future greatness, – been educated beyond my fortunes – and formed tastes, and cherished feelings, incompatible with the station it seems I was born to – beggary or daily labour!'[84] In essence, he has attempted to transcend his social class and is now suffering his punishment. While the late physician sympathises with his plight, noting that a 'keen recollection of similar scenes in my own history, almost brought the tears into my eyes', he is shocked by his patient's haughty refusal of the sacrament.[85] His discontented death, haunted by 'fearful thoughts',[86] contrasts markedly with the godly deathbed scenes of the physician's more pious patients in chapters such as 'The Martyr-Philosopher' and 'The Magdalen', whose highly sentimentalised, peaceful death from consumption is precipitated by her atonement for falling prey to a vivacious and false suitor far above her social station. She dies doubly thankful for the mercy of God and the goodness of the physician, who has saved her from dying disgraced in a brothel. Before relaying her tale, the 'editor' declares to the reader: 'Many as are the scenes of guilt and misery sketched in this Diary, I know not that I have approached any with feelings of such profound and unmixed sorrow as that which it is my painful lot now to lay before the public.' He encourages his readers, however, to let their own tears 'swell into a stream' – to think on the story of 'The Magdalen' and then dare try and become a corruptor of innocent virtue.[87]

Medical Morality: John Gregory's Medical Ethics

The late physician's status as a medical man of feeling is vital to the explicit morality of the series. In the tradition of moral sense philosophy, prominent in Scotland following the influential work of Francis Hutchinson, 'natural' feelings were viewed as the common arbiter of right and wrong for all mankind, and in Gregory's system of medical ethics, the medical practitioner was particularly obliged to remain attentive to the sentiments of sympathy and humanity as guides to moral action.[88] As Robert Baker explains, in *Lectures on the Duties and Qualifications of a Physician*, Gregory 'characterizes "humanity" as "that sensibility of heart which makes us feel for the distresses of our fellow creatures, and which of a consequence, incites us to relieve them"', while '[s]ympathy is the sentiment which engages the humanity of the moral practitioner and makes it operational by "produc[ing] an anxious attention to a thousand little circumstances that may tend to relieve the patient"'.[89] According to Laurence B. McCullough, Gregory followed Hume's declaration that 'Reason is, and ought only to be the slave of the passions' in discussing the ideal moral physician, while Lisbeth Haakonssen views Gregory as responding more generally to notions of sympathy current in the late eighteenth century, extending to the Common Sense philosophers.[90]

Regardless of the roots of his ideas, Gregory clearly explains the key place of the feelings in medical practice:

> The faculty has often been reproached with hardness of heart, occasioned, as is supposed, but [sic] their being so much conversant with human misery. I hope and believe the charge is unjust; for habit may beget a command of temper, and a seeming composure, which is often mistaken for absolute insensibility. But, by the way, I must observe, that, when this insensibility is real, it is an misfortune to a physician, as it deprives him of one of the most natural and powerful incitements to exert himself for the relief of his patient.[91]

Gregory does warn against an excessive sensibility to distress, since

> a physician of too much sensibility may be rendered incapable of doing
> his duty from anxiety, and excess of sympathy, which cloud his under-
> standing, depress his spirit, and prevent him from acting with that
> steadiness and vigour, upon which perhaps the life of his patient in a
> great measure depends.[92]

Balance was the ideal, and Moir's critique of the series as 'overdrawn'
is indicative of Warren's transgressions. However, the late physician's
sensibility is frequently redeemed through its function as the underlying motive for humane action. In 'A Scholar's Death-Bed', for example, the physician's sympathetic feelings motivate him to sustain the
scholar from 'literal starvation',[93] while his ability to 'enter into every
feeling' of the virtuous yet destitute and ailing couple in 'The Merchant's Clerk' leads him to attempt to intervene in their situation.[94]
Their destitution is a result of the young woman's father, Mr Hilary,
having disowned her for marrying his clerk:

> It was after listening to one of the most interesting and melancholy
> narratives that the annals of human suffering could supply, that I
> secretly resolved to take upon myself the responsibility of appealing
> to Mr Hilary in their behalf, hoping that for the honour of humanity
> my efforts would not be entirely unavailing.[95]

'[M]oved to action' by his patient's narrative, the late physician
seems to exemplify not only Gregory's moral physician but also a
nineteenth-century practitioner of Rita Charon's twenty-first-century
'Narrative Medicine'.[96]

The 'ideal of the humanistic physician' may be a 'commonplace
today';[97] however, Gregory's text was highly innovative in the late
eighteenth century and responded to key challenges faced by medical
practitioners.[98] The crisis of faith in the aristocratic honour codes
that had previously guided doctor–patient relationships necessitated a behavioural code that transcended a simple appeal to polite
manners.[99] If texts such as the Earl of Chesterfield's letters to his son,
published in 1774, revealed that 'good manners were not so much
the sign of innate virtue as the indicator of social expediency', how
was the physician to establish credibility?[100] Additionally, with the

growing demand for medical services, how was the profession to distinguish itself from the self-interestedness of capitalist trade?[101] Gregory's appeal to moral sense philosophy provided the answer, as medical morality became a development of character and a function of constant attentiveness to one's own motivations.[102] Those who followed Gregory's advice were to take care that their motivation remained rooted in sympathy and humanity, as social ambition and desire for pecuniary reward could only lead to the production of false (i.e. affected) sympathy.[103] According to Warren's preface to the People's Edition, his series provided a key service to the medical profession in depicting this motivation for a popular audience – in attempting 'to awaken society to a sense of its incalculable obligations to Medical Men' and to portray '[t]he amount of misery and suffering which they alleviate, cheerfully and patiently, often altogether gratuitously'.[104] While the 'Early Struggles' focuses on the late physician's desperate need for pecuniary reward, throughout the remainder of the series we witness the physician delicately refusing fees and expressing his social duty to minister to all.

But does the late physician really portray the type of 'disciplined engagement with distress and loss' advocated by Gregory and his nineteenth-century successors?[105] According to McCullough, a key aspect of the ethical relationship described by Gregory was the privileging of the patient's interests such that the physician might become obligated to 'do something disagreeable, i.e., *against* the physician's interest'.[106] In this formulation, Gregory added '*moral* authority' to the '*intellectual* and *clinical* authority' of the physician.[107] Warren's series – with its Johnsonian motto – appears explicitly to build upon this authority, and the case of 'A "Man About Town"' is perhaps the best example of the late physician's actively working to quell self-interest for the sake of a patient. However, the tale also clearly exemplifies the series' rather less disinterested participation in the commercial vogue for voyeuristic, sensational tales, which, as will be discussed later in this chapter, was a tension that the series' critics highlighted.

In 'A "Man About Town"', the physician's emotive reaction is not exquisite sorrow but rather repulsion as he cares for the rakish debauchee, Henry Effingstone, who suffers a torturously slow demise from syphilis. (The disease is unnamed yet implied through lurid descriptions of his gnawing bone pains, putrid rotting flesh, and progressive mental alienation.) The physician waits upon the once fashionable and wealthy young man in a common boarding house, far below his station; at Effingstone's fervent insistence he promises to keep his patient's illness and location secret, despite his knowledge that 'in the event of any thing sudden befalling him, the censure of all his relatives would be levelled at me'.[108] The horrors of the sickroom progressively tell on the physician, and he affirms:

> I think I can say with truth and sincerity, that scarce the wealth of the Indies should tempt me to undertake the management of another such case. I am losing my appetite – loathe animal food – am haunted day and night by the piteous spectacle which I have to encounter daily in Mr Effingstone.[109]

Nurses and landladies desert Effingstone; his oldest friend – the one individual to whom he calls out – refuses to see him; and yet the late physician and Effingstone's loyal servant, George, remain by his side.

In his lectures Gregory was also keen to counteract the common accusations of scepticism and infidelity levelled against the medical profession, and those who built upon his work in the early nineteenth century, such as Thomas Percival, Sir Benjamin Brodie, John Abercrombie, and Sir Henry Halford, continued to emphasise the Christian duties of the medical man.[110] Following this broader movement, in addition to his increasingly futile medical treatments, the late physician also attempts to minister to Effingstone's soul, and Effingstone thus characteristically becomes a moral as well as a medical case study. The physician is at first puzzled that one so gifted 'as to intellect' may yet possess a soul apparently 'utterly destitute of any sympathies for virtue', but identifies the 'key to his character' when he overhears Effingstone's father refer to him as 'a *splendid* sinner'.[111] He reasons that the 'placid approval of virtue' would be 'infinitely less stimulating to his morbid sensibilities' than his 'Satanic satisfaction in the consciousness of being an object of regret and wonder among those who most enthusiastically acknowledged his intellectual supremacy'.[112] Standing at the precipice of his darkest hours of illness, Effingstone casts off the physician's attempts to provide religious consolation and insists that the 'tried disciplined energies' of his own mind will sustain him through his sufferings.[113] The horrific derangement and demonic visions that follow reveal the failure of his mental powers, and his case becomes an exemplar of the type of scene that Gregory thought predisposed the physician towards religion. The physician, Gregory writes,

> has many opportunities of seeing people, once the gay and the happy, sunk in deep distress; sometimes devoted to a painful and lingering death; and sometimes struggling with the tortures of a distracted mind. Such afflictive scenes, one should imagine, might soften any heart not dead to every feeling of humanity, and make it reverence that religion which alone can support the soul in the most complicated distresses; that religion, which teaches to enjoy life with cheerfulness, and to resign it with dignity.[114]

However, religion does not support the soul of the 'Man About Town', whose habitual blasphemy – now 'bred in the bone' – cannot even be overcome in a brief moment of 'bettered feelings'.[115] He finds not consolation but rather assured damnation in any religious reflections. His unrepentant depravity is engrained into his mind and body, as his 'detestable debauchery' has, according to the late physician, 'vitiated and depraved his whole system, both physical and mental'.[116]

Habit was central to Gregory's medical ethics and to those who followed him, and Effingstone may be read as a case study of what the moral physician in the Scottish tradition should never be. According to Percival,

> no profession is more favourable, than that of physic, to the formation of a mental constitution, which unites in it very high degrees of intellectual and moral vigour; because it calls forth the steady and unremitting exertions of benevolence, under the direction of cultivated reason; and, by opening a wider and wider sphere of duty, progressively augments their reciprocal energies.[117]

However, if individuals pervert this natural connection through 'coldness of heart' and 'a sceptical turn of thinking', 'virtuous principles will gradually decay; all tender charities of life will soon be extinguished; a future state will be either disbelieved or regarded with indifference; and practical atheism will ensue, with the whole train of evils which result from a denial of the creative agency of God, or his divine administration'.[118] In his *Inquiries Concerning the Intellectual Powers and the Investigation of Truth*, Abercrombie writes that

> [t]his condition of mind presents a subject of intense interest, to every one who would study his own mental condition, either as an intellectual or a moral being. In each individual instance, it may be traced to a particular course of thought and of conduct, by which the mind went gradually more and more astray from truth and from virtue. In this progress, each single step was felt to be a voluntary act; but the influence of the whole, after a certain period, is to distort the judgment, and deaden the moral feelings on the great questions of truth and rectitude.[119]

For Abercrombie, the only cure for this state of moral depravity is the Christian redemption that Effingstone repeatedly rejects.

The late physician, in contrast, in writing the case of 'A "Man About Town"', is performing the very type of mental exercise recommended by Abercrombie to promote moral and intellectual rectitude. In his chapter on a 'Well-regulated mind' he writes 'that our condition, in the scale both of moral and intellectual beings is, in a great measure, determined by the control which we have acquired over the succession of our thoughts, and by the subjects on which they are habitually exercised',[120] and in a later edition he further recommends the 'habit of following out a connected chain of thought on subjects of importance and of truth, whenever the mind is disengaged from the proper and necessary attention to the ordinary transactions of life'.[121] In writing up his diary of memorable cases, the late physician enables both himself and the reader to clearly view the posited causal relations between vice, disease and even death. In such acts, moral authority becomes inextricability linked to narrative authority.

Narrative Authority: The Literary Late Physician

In Chapter 2, I discussed the Blackwoodian tale of terror as a critical inversion of the case histories that appeared in the *Edinburgh Monthly Magazine*, as the subject of the physical or psychological trauma, rather than an authoritative observer, comes to narrate the experience. Warren's series represents a return to the physician-as-narrator of the case history, and like Howison and Macnish, who also developed the tale of terror in this direction, he maintains the characteristic embodied subjectivity of the narrative voice, and thus includes a polemical emotive and aesthetic dimension to the epistemic genre of the case history. The physician himself experiences trauma as he is alternately repulsed, terrified, and sympathetically moved by his patients. To provide just one more example: in the case of 'The Forger', the late physician is called to attend a young gentleman, a 'Mr Gloucester', who appears to be suffering from a nervous malady. The true cause for his mental uneasiness is revealed when 'two sullen Newgate myrmidons' come to arrest him for forgery.[122] Both the physician and the patient's responses are melodramatically recorded:

> I rose from my chair, and staggered a few paces, I knew not whither. I could scarce preserve myself from falling on the floor. Mr. Gloucester, as soon as he caught sight of the officers, fell back on the ottoman – suddenly pressed his hand to his heart – turned pale as death, and gasped, breathless with horror.[123]

When Gloucester is finally hanged for his crime, the tale focuses on the response of the physician, who witnesses the execution from a house 'immediately opposite the gloomy gallows', rather than on the traumatic experience of the sufferer, as in the tale of 'Le Revenant':

> I staggered from my place at the window to a distant part of the room, dropped into a chair, shut my eyes, closed my tingling ears with my fingers, – and, with a hurried aspiration for God's mercy toward the wretched young criminal who, within a very few yards of me, was, perhaps, that instant surrendering his life into the hands which gave it.[124]

Scenes such as these lead Kennedy to conclude that the late physician endangered 'the professional standing of the physician by insisting on his subjective embodiment rather than his rational, distanced perspective'.[125]

However, the late physician, like the authoritative narrators of the early case histories discussed in Chapter 2, is also a collector of traumatic narratives, and it is he, rather than the patient, who has control over how the narrative is crafted and presented. 'Editorial' footnotes, ever multiplying through subsequent editions, confirm his authority by providing a range of parallel cases, and his control is repeatedly emphasised to the reader. For example, at the opening of 'The Spectre-Smitten', the physician notes that 'I have not given the *whole* of my observations – far from it; those only are recorded which seemed to me to have some claims to consideration of both medical and general readers'.[126] In 'The Wife' he acknowledges that he has received the narrative from 'the reluctant lips of the poor sufferer herself', but then declares that he must 'be allowed to give it in my own way' and promises to 'conclude with extracting some portions of my notes of visits made in a professional capacity'.[127] Warren's particular use of the generic mode of the tale of terror manages to highlight the late physician's sensibility and his professional authority both together. As Howard Brody observes, '[p]hysicians, because of their knowledge and their social role, have special powers to construct stories and to persuade others that these stories are the true stories of the illness'.[128] These powers are not unique to the twentieth century: perhaps since Hippocrates the physician's authority has been linked to authorship. Warren simply made this more visible to a popular audience.

Throughout the series the late physician is presented as a highly competent reader and writer of his patient's narratives. In his introduction to 'The Ruined Merchant' he reflects that while '[p]oor stupid unobserving man' often 'cannot conceive how it comes to pass that all the evils under the run are showered down upon *his* head – at once', in most such cases 'a ready solution may be found, by any one of observation'.[129] In this case the 'ready solution' is the 'peculiar perils incident to rapidly acquired fortune, which often lifts its possessor into an element for which he is totally unfitted'. The late physician traces causal links between commercial speculation, growing insatiable desire for wealth, and family ruin in a case that at once critiques the commercial spirit and reifies the 'natural' laws of high Tory ideology.[130]

The physician's keen reading abilities are also revealed by his particular way of writing the case, which often reconstructs his detection of the causal chain. The most poignant example of this is perhaps 'The Spectre-Smitten', which opens by identifying the immediate cause of Mr M—'s madness (extreme fright at seeing the spectre of his deceased neighbour) and then follows the late physician's initial unravelling of the case as it progresses from an apparent epileptic fit to the extremes of violent madness and eventual suicide. The physician only comes to fully understand the cause of his patient's sudden mental illness when he takes on the role of amanuensis for Mr M— during his ravings, and identifies 'one individual image of horror' that recurs in 'various similar expressions and allusions': that of 'a "*dark parlour, with some fiery-faced fiend sitting in an arm-chair*"'.[131] This is, of course, the spectral image that the reader knows Mr M— experienced just before the onset of his madness. Further, Mr M—'s madness is marked by a desire to write a romance, and the late physician identifies the style of Charles Maturin in his incoherent writings: the same author whose works of diablerie are said to fascinate Mr M— at the opening of the case, predisposing his mind to spectral visions. Mr M—'s incompetent exercises in fiction contrast starkly with the late physician's narrative mastery; health becomes associated with the realist discourse of the case history, and disease with the pathological imagination of Gothic romance. A footnote amended to the first edition further authorises this reading: 'Since this was published, I have been favoured by Sir Henry Halford, with the sight of a narrative of a case remarkably similar to the present one, but told, I need hardly say, with far more graphic ability.'[132]

Sir Henry Halford, president of the Royal College of Physicians of London from 1820 until his death in 1844, was a major advocate of 'narrative competence' (to evoke Charon's terminology) and also shared Warren's fascination with deathbed scenes. In today's parlance 'narrative competence' refers to a higher level of attentiveness to a patient's particular story – an ability 'to recognize, absorb, interpret, and be moved by the stories of illness' – in an effort to counter the current reductionism of biomedicine.[133] However, in the context of nineteenth-century British medicine, narrative ability asserted the authoritative power of the medical professional. Halford's *On the Deaths of some Eminent Persons of Modern Times* (1835), first delivered at the RCP and subsequently published by Murray, contains perhaps his most overt statement of the narrative authority of physicians. At the close of this oration, he entreats the reader to read history

> with some mistrust and reserve, recollecting how difficult it is to develope [sic] the motives of human conduct; how easily the spirit of party insinuates itself into the historian's mind, and colours his narrative;

and how almost impossible it is for an unprofessional writer to appreciate fully the effect of diseases of the body upon the minds and actions of men.[134]

The professional physician, however, is granted the ability to authorise a more authentic narrative, and Halford provides several examples, including explanations of the behaviour of 'eminent' figures such as Dean Swift and George II shortly before their deaths, emphasising the links between their mental states and bodily disease and verifying his readings via the results of post-mortem examinations. While the late physician provides an authoritative narrative of exemplary individual cases, distinguishing normative narrative abilities from the pathological, in this oration Halford attempts the grander project of providing authoritative historical and biographical narratives, looking forward to the twentieth- and twenty-first-century practice of 'retrospective diagnosis' – the bane of today's medical historians and medical humanists alike.

Halford was an associate of Warren's in London, and the fourth and fifth editions of the *Diary* were dedicated to him following Warren's suggestion to Alexander Blackwood that it would 'aid the vraisemblance of the thing – as being dedicated to the first physician of the age'.[135] Halford's name, however, was first associated with Warren's series by an article in the *London Medical Gazette*, which accuses him of borrowing 'Sir Henry Halford's elegant illustration of a passage in Shakspeare [sic] . . . without scruple or acknowledgment'.[136] The passage referred to is 'Hamlet's test of sanity – the *re-wording of the matter*', cited in Warren's 'Intriguing and Madness' as

Bring me to the test,
And I *the matter will re-word*, which *madness*
Would gambol from.[137]

In an address to the RCP, reported in the *London Medical Gazette* in June 1829, Halford illustrated the utility and accuracy of Hamlet's test in a case from his own practice, and Warren similarly equates narrative incompetence with mental derangement in 'Intriguing and Madness' when he has a deranged young man cite Hamlet's test (attributing it incorrectly to *King Lear*) and then fail it by immediately losing his ability 'to take up the chain of his thoughts'.[138]

Halford's reputation provides some insight into the mixed reception of the late physician, which will be explored in the following sections by looking at some key parodies and imitations. As president of the RCP and as a tireless defender of the value of a classical education, Halford was by no means universally esteemed.[139] To advocates of medical reform he represented everything that was wrong with the elite practitioners who sought to maintain their dominance against the inevitability of progress. According to *The Lancet*, '[h]e is all tact and nothing else. He is ignorant of the modern discoveries in pathology and never employs the modern instruments of diagnosis; he has never written a line that is worthy of perusal on any scientific subject.'[140] While *The Lancet* was known to be harshly vindictive towards political opponents, in his *On the Education and Conduct of a Physician* (1834) Halford does advise medical students not to pay too much attention to chemistry, botany, and anatomy, and he focuses instead upon the importance of moral development through classical education and upon manners. Most problematically, in an age in which the display of good manners was no certain indicator of moral worth, Halford places rather too much emphasis on self-interested results rather than on internal motivation. He notes that 'sensibility and tenderness' will 'be likely to conciliate the sick man's confidence and attachment' and should be extended to the family around the sickbed as well, since 'the impression [such conduct] makes will be remembered and acknowledged by future confidence and esteem'.[141] In his 1772 lectures, Gregory had advised that one may determine false from genuine sympathy by seeing how physicians treat their inferiors and persons from whom they have nothing to gain.[142] Contemporary accounts indicate that Halford failed this test miserably.[143]

Perhaps unsurprisingly, Warren's late physician was criticised for mirroring some aspects of elite medical culture. As we will see in the following sections, the parodies and imitations that followed often take up this theme. However, one of the most fascinating aspects of the *Diary* is that regardless of – and perhaps even because of – such criticisms, the series prompted others to take up their pens and build upon Warren's medico-popular representation of the medical profession.

Parody in the Periodicals

In January 1831 the *New Monthly Magazine* announced that '[a] SUDDEN partiality appears to incline the fashionable and literary world towards the mysteries of the healing art'. The author of the anonymous article notes a distinctive shift: 'Physic is no longer thrown to the dogs by our Modern Shakespeares.'[144] Marking a key moment in the transition from Georgian satire to Victorian idealisation, Warren's series captured the popular and professional imagination alike and prompted numerous parodies and imitations. Following Warren's model, this emergent generic hybrid featured first-person narration by a medical practitioner, which often blended autobiography with the case history form, and was characterised by an insistent realism that included appeals to physical records such as diaries and notebooks, as well as recalled experiences in the form of 'sketches' or 'reminiscences'. These texts frequently echo Warren's celebration of the medical practitioner as uniquely positioned to record domestic dramas, to observe human character unveiled and thus to provide moral insight into the human condition,[145] and they also range from overt didacticism to Gothic horror and humorous adventure story. Particularly in the immediate aftermath of the series' publication, they at times consciously critique or authoritatively correct Warren's portrayal of the late physician. Like the original *Diary*, several of these texts emerge from the politicised forum of the popular periodical press.

The quotation regarding the literary vogue for the healing art, cited above, comes from the opening of an early parody of Warren's series, 'Some Passages from the Diary of a Late Fashionable Apothecary', which appeared in the *New Monthly* in January 1831. It is no tribute to the late physician of *Blackwood's*. Rather, the parody amplifies the satire that 'Early Struggles' may have achieved had it been published in the *New Monthly*. The 'late fashionable apothecary' is a doting product of the peerage, rather than a Cambridge man attempting to make it in the cutthroat London medical marketplace. He declares that 'I cannot, like my eminent coadjutor of Blackwood's, prevail on myself to accuse the harshness of my early fortunes.'[146] Raised within the household of the Earl of Worthing, the darling son of two favoured domestics, the apothecary has been trained from the start to curry patronage from his social superiors, 'to simper under an affront, and return bow for blow'.[147] His unabashed sycophancy, coming from an apothecary rather than a physician, amplifies the vulgarity of his ludicrous displays, and he lays the foundation for his practice not through a legitimate medical encounter but rather by attempting to save the favourite pugs of the Dowager from being poisoned by her grandson, Lord Lancing, who, in fact, never intended to poison them at all. At first insulted that the apothecary could think her grandson capable of such criminality, the Dowager is won over when the apothecary seizes one of the pugs and 'bade him put up his innocent paws in my behalf, even as the youthful Dauphin of France was taught to intercede for Marie-Antoinette with the Parisian popu-lace!' He declares his success:

> This little *ruse* was successful: my excess of zeal was first pardoned, and at length commended. From that hour I date the overflowing patronage of the Dowager, and my own fortunes. *Within a year, I became master of a chariot – and a wife!*[148]

Competence is questionable – but competence is not required for professional success. The apothecary, and by proxy, the late phy-sician are both associated with the 'cringing pulse-feeling race' earlier decried by the *New Monthly*, while the apothecary's ridicu-lously florid language and melodramatic descriptions of mundane events emphasise the superficiality and narcissism that mark the 'fashionable' practitioner.

Fraser's was even more overt in its parody. At first blush, one might find it out of keeping with the magazine's avowed politics to find anything offensive in the *Diary*.[149] While refusing to align itself directly with either the Whig or Tory parties in their opening 'Con-fession of Faith' of February 1830, the magazine was conservative in the model of Coleridge and Southey – defenders of Church and State – and certainly 'not of *liberal* principles'.[150] Even as late as March 1848, at which point the magazine became more liberal under the management of the William John Parkers,[151] an article entitled 'A Plea for Physicians' laments the competition that well-educated physicians were facing from both GPs and apothecaries by the 1840s, and argues that reform must reassert the authority of traditionally well-educated men: laissez-faire economics must not be allowed to destroy the noble profession.[152] However, the late physician became a target in *Fraser's* for two important reasons: the attack was part of a struggle to dethrone Maga as the 'Queen of Literary Magazines'[153] as well as of a much wider attempt to diagnose the degeneracy of British literary culture,[154] which, in the Fraserian context, was paralleled by the degeneracy of British medicine.

In their 'Notices to Correspondents' in August 1830, *Fraser's* responds to a request that the 'odious quackery' of the *Diary* be exposed in their pages. They firmly refuse: 'The dulness [sic] and frippery, the base coinage of lead and dross in exhausted Magazines do not fall within the peculiar province of our administration of critical law.'[155] 'Quack' and 'quackery' are slippery terms to pin down in the early nineteenth century,[156] but within the early numbers of *Fraser's* they are used to refer to persons and actions which are all pretence and no substance, and which falsely claim disinterestedness, talent and learning while preying upon the credulity of the masses for financial gain. One of the greatest transgressors, according to *Fraser's*, was the fashionable novelist Edward Bulwer-Lytton.[157]

Such behaviour plagued both the literary and medical industries in the period that saw the rise of a mass-market economy. In April 1830 William Maginn denounced Henry Colburn as the 'Prince Paramount of Puffers and Quacks' for using periodicals he owned to advertise and provide favourable reviews of books he published and sold,[158] and the following month, in a piece 'On Medical Quackery and Mr. St. John Long', attributed to Thomas Carlyle's brother, John Aitken Carlyle, the magazine announces: 'We have declared open war against all quacks, of whatsoever sort, and shall always be ready at our post, using all the means in our power to set them forth in their true light, and bring them into their proper places.'[159] In this and two articles to follow, John St John Long (1798–1834) of Harley Street, who was frequently declared a 'quack' by his contemporaries, is derided as avaricious and affected.[160] The public could be easily fooled, but *Fraser's* avowed to unveil hypocrisy and, at least in the domain of literature, set appropriate critical standards.[161]

Warren's series appears to have fallen rather below these standards. According to *Fraser's* response in the 'Notices to Correspondents', its 'false sentiment and beastly detail' – its 'clothing' of 'brothel-thoughts in tawdry language' – makes exposure of it unnecessary: 'it is transparent, and all behold the vile deformity beneath'.[162] However, the popularity of the *Diary* persisted,[163] and the January 1831 number of *Fraser's* contains a parody that does the supposedly unnecessary. In the aptly named 'Some Passages from the Diary of the late Mr. St. John Long', Long boasts of the 'ample fee-licity' he finds in alleviating suffering and relates his witnessing of 'a spectacle of the most appalling character'.[164] His attempted treatment of an unconscious patient he believes to be suffering from '*phthilis pulmonalis*' culminates in ludicrous melodrama, as the patient's 'aged nurse' with 'the tear of affection' glistening in her eye, vomits in response to his remedies. In the end it transpires that the patient had simply been '*drunk the night before*', and in a rage at the quack's attempted treatment he chases him out of the house, launching a 'curious crown of crockery' at his head which 'fitted on so tightly' that only by 'breaking it' does Long 'disengage' himself from the 'delphic diadem'.[165] Florid and often alliterative language masks toilet humour, and the implication is simple: like the medical quack, Warren's series is fraudulent – a 'hollow-hearted' display of extravagance, crude voyeurism and sentiment intended to attract readers.[166] However, through its obvious vulgarity it instead repulses them. Even the drunkard knows well enough to throw the physician out of the house.

Warren found *Fraser's* parody slightly ironic. Like many of *Blackwood's* notable contributors, he was offered large sums of money to defect from his position as '"Physician" to the regiment' of 'the corps of Sir Christopher' and instead become a 'Fraserian'.[167] He reports offers of as much as £40 and £50 per chapter of the *Diary*, while Blackwood paid him only £20.[168] According to Patrick Leary's account of the magazine's early financial management, high sums were offered to writers whose work promised high returns (though not even Thomas Carlyle was paid as much as Warren claims to have been offered): so much for *Fraser's* critique of the physician's 'fee-licity'.[169] However, *Fraser's* may have felt some satisfaction in September 1832 when they were able to report the true quackery of the series – that the author of the *Diary* was 'a young London barrister' who has merely 'personated the physician with sufficient accuracy to pass as such with the mass of readers'. They are careful to point out, however, that 'of course, medical people will see at once that he is not one of themselves'.[170]

Moir and Macnish's letters indicate the veracity of their conclusion. Try as he might, Warren did not get it quite right. However, what was 'right' was in flux, and where one might place the late physician on the sliding scale between ideal moral and religious medico-literary figure and fashionable quack depended largely on one's political stance and literary allegiance. Regardless of whether it posed a threat to some ideals of medical professionalism or depicted a form of medical humanism likely to win not a few admirers, the series opened up a much wider conversation about the struggles of medical life and provided a model for actual medical practitioners with literary ambitions to imitate.

The Real Physicians' Diaries

The relationship between the medical profession and the wider public became a key theme of the writings of the actual medical practitioners who followed Warren's model, and a primary concern appears to have been that the late physician catered to the elite rather than to the growing middle- and even working-class market. *The Doctor, A Medical Magazine* (1833–8) contains a particularly explicit example in 'The Real Diary of a Physician'. Apparently ignoring Warren's depictions of extreme deprivation in 'Rich and Poor' and 'The Magdalen', a prefatory article of April 1833 declares that the series was clearly written for and about the 'opulent' and thus 'wore the air of melo-drama rather than the stern realities of life'.[171] Their 'real' diary promises to provide the 'authentic history of the rise and progress of a physician' and thus 'exhibit in glowing colours the wrongs that the medical profession sustains at the hands of the public, and on the other part the injustice that the public suffers from the profession'.[172] Their proposed agenda of acting as arbitrators between the equally wronged profession and general public is unrealised, however, as only one number follows – a more mundane and less emotive rendition of the 'Early Struggles', which relates how a young surgeon-apothecary (who does go on to become a physician in London, despite his dislike for the RCP) establishes himself by accidentally saving the child of a local minister from choking. The message is essentially the same as that which opens Johnson's 'Life of Akenside' in *Lives of the Most Eminent English Poets* (1779–81): that public favour is utterly unrelated to true ability.

Macmichael's *Golden-Headed Cane* (1827), the subsequent multi-authored *Lives of British Physicians* (1830), and Forbes Winslow's

Physic and Physicians: A Medical Sketch Book, Exhibiting the Public and Private Life of the most Celebrated Medical Men, Of Former Days; With Memoirs of Eminent Living London Physicians and Surgeons (1839) all take their prompt from Johnson's suggestion that 'a very curious book might be written on the "Fortune of Physicians"'.[173] However, Warren's particular model, when followed through at least, enabled something that medical biography could not provide – an apparent window into the internal motivations and reactions, the feelings and thoughts that the public could not normally see. One of the most successful texts in this mode, Alexander Maxwell Adams's *Sketches from Life. By a Physician* (1835), fully exploits this potential to dramatic effect.

At the time *Sketches* was published, Adams was a GP in Edinburgh, though he would go on to gain his M.D. and found a 'dynasty of doctors' culminating in a writer, Douglas Adams (1952–2001), author of *The Hitch-Hiker's Guide to the Galaxy*.[174] In the Preface Maxwell Adams claims that 'some years have now passed since many of the observations, contained in the following sheets, were first committed to paper' and insists that the appearance of what he terms 'Extracts from the Diary of a Physician' has delayed rather than prompted publication of his work.[175] If this is the case, then Scottish medical men were more generally reflecting upon the role of the moral feelings in medical practice at this time. The first tale in the volume, 'The Curate's Daughter; or, The Victim of Irish Anarchy and English Despotism', which draws upon Adams's Ulster heritage, is based upon the physician following out the 'impulse of feeling' to assist a dying young woman and her child, and thus providentially to complete an act of benevolent self-sacrifice from many years prior.[176] The woman recalls his previous aid, describing how the physician 'felt with me, and for me', and in their reunion the physician notes that he again 'entered deeply into her feelings'.[177] When he succeeds in providing for her orphaned daughter by forcing her malevolent estranged father to acknowledge her birthright, his feelings well up uncontrollably the moment he is left alone: 'I felt my heart grow womanish, and in spite of all the stoicism that either my philosophy or my intercourse with society had taught me, I wept like a child.'[178]

Adams, however, also reflects on the accompanying risks of unregulated sensibility in medical practice, an issue largely ignored by Warren. In 'The Casuist; or, Delineations and Observations of a Sentimentalist', the longest tale of Adams's volume, his patient is a fellow-physician who is bankrupt and dying under 'the influence of a too sensitive mind'.[179] The patient's hypersensitivity and his financial straits are linked to his early classical education: D'Albert has 'devoted the early and best portion of his life to the acquirement of knowledge, which in his subsequent life afforded him no adequate return'.[180] D'Albert is considered no singular example, and his case prompts Adams to reflect upon the flawed process of medical education. After being raised on the classics, the 'finer feelings' of the student are 'seared by a practical use of the dissecting knife'.[181] Then, the young medical man finds that what he has learned is not necessarily advantageous in the medical marketplace, where he is 'surrounded by jealous contemporaries and jaundiced rivals, ready to cripple the advances of merit, and discourage the exertions of ingenuous worth'.[182] In the end, he realises that public appearance – his perceived worth – is everything, and he must 'war with his own nature' to get ahead.[183]

D'Albert spurns such ingratiations – writing pamphlets against the corruption of a society that turns natural benevolence into selfishness – and the public turns against him. Adams, however, views himself as a medico-literary middleman of sorts, occupying a space between the world of imagination and fine feelings occupied by literary men such as D'Albert and that of common men, who 'are occupied with the things of this life only, and enjoy themselves in their own unscientific way'.[184] He muses, 'My qualifications and pursuits being intermediate of these two conditions, I could, to an extent feel with both,'[185] and in writing his *Sketches*, as one of a 'highly-privileged and enlightened class', he attempts to bring his literary abilities to bear on common life.[186] In his subsequent lament that so few other medical men have followed suit, Adams echoes Moir and Macnish's statements regarding the contemporary reception of literary medical men, and lays the blame on the British public and their prejudices against

> the name of 'an author': the half-lettered and illiterate, which compose the great bulk of people, considering it incompatible with professional dignity, and a sufficient pretext for withholding or withdrawing their patronage from the fool-hardy wight who bears it.[187]

However, as these varied imitations illustrate, Warren's series had initiated a generic model well adapted for the professional medical man
of the nineteenth century. It hinged upon the relationship between
medical, moral and narrative authority, and through its medico-literary hybridity occupied the already established realm of medical
writing, drawing upon clinical realism and the case history tradition,
while also allowing for more reflexive and familiar commentary and
literary experimentation.

Both the *Monthly* and the *New Monthly Magazine* soon refor-
mulated their medico-popular articles to follow Warren's model.
'Experiences of a Surgeon', which ran through five numbers in the
Monthly in 1835, contains echoes of the tale of terror, portraying,
for example, a young surgeon's dramatic struggle with a madman
and 'A Dissecting-Room Incident' in which the surgeon vividly
describes the 'most singular and extraordinary feelings' he experiences when he believes the half-decayed corpses have come back to
life and formed a 'Frankenstein'.[188] However, it also carries forward
the careful detailing of medical cases from the discontinued 'Medical
Report' series, containing a greater specificity of clinical knowledge
than Warren's series, while at the same time emphasising the surgeon's compassion for his patients. In turn, the *New Monthly* subsequently published a series of six 'Extracts' or 'Sketches from the
Note-book of a Physician' between October 1839 and August 1840,
written by the Edinburgh physician Anthony Todd Thomson (1778–
1849). The series provides medical information on topics such as
hypochondria, consumption, insanity and the dangers of London
air, in a mode suited to a general audience, illustrated by exemplary
cases and delivered by a benevolent yet dignified physician narrator,
keen to highlight the latest medical advances, including, most notably, the stethoscope.[189] 'Reminiscences of a Medical Student', written by the Glaswegian naval surgeon Robert Douglas (b. 1820) and
published in the *New Monthly* from December 1841 to April 1844,
moves in the opposite direction, providing a series of sensational
adventure stories with little genuine medical information. Instead,
his 'Reminiscences' look nostalgically back to earlier in the century
and work against the assumption that the man of science must be 'a
cold, grave, abstracted being, unwitting of the creature-comforts of
this life'.[190] Ever adaptable and dynamically evolving, however, the

genre responded to progressive medical developments and the ever-changing struggles of medical life.

None of the actual medical practitioners who followed Warren's model, whom I have identified to date, truly rival the sensibility of the late physician, and the balance between the feelings and the intellect appears to have been consciously recalibrated.[191] However, the genre clearly maintained its humanist potential. A key example is Dr John Brown's 'Rab and His Friends', first published in 1858 but based on his experience as an apprentice at Minto House surgical hospital in December 1830. Echoing Warren's 'Cancer', Brown sentimentally depicts a woman's heroism in undergoing a painful mastectomy, again, prior to the advent of anaesthesia, focusing on her ability to touch even the hardening hearts of young medical students. The students observing the procedure are at first only concerned with obtaining a good view and understanding the medical details of the case. Brown excuses their apparent inhumanity:

> Don't think them heartless; they are neither better nor worse than you or I; they get over their professional horrors, and into their proper work; and in them pity – as an *emotion*, ending in itself or at best in tears and a long-drawn breath, lessens, while pity, as a *motive*, is quickened, and gains power and purpose. It is well for poor human nature that it is so.[192]

However, the appearance of the patient silences the students' irreverent chattering: 'These rough boys feel the power of her presence', and her gentle submissiveness during the surgical procedure and her apology to the crowd afterwards, begging 'pardon if she has behaved ill', causes all of the medical students to weep 'like children'.[193]

The Political Late Physician

From Arthur Conan Doyle's *Round the Red Lamp* (1894) and the medical short stories of William Carlos Williams (1883–1963) to A. J. Cronin's Dr Finlay tales (adapted for radio and television by the BBC), Warren's model has continued to evolve with the times. However, in the context of the turbulent 1830s, Warren's series had particular political salience. His depiction of a gentlemanly physician-figure clearly works against the ideals of those who sought to eliminate medical hierarchies through medical reform, but the series' emphasis on the moral duty and privilege of the medical profession, and the humane motivations ideally behind the practice of medicine, also speaks more broadly to the profession's growing collective identity at this time.

One of the key issues that united the medical profession in this period was a general sense of dissatisfaction with the New Poor Law of 1834, which infamously strove to manage medical provision for the poor in England according to Malthusian principles.[194] Not only did the New Poor Law raise the standards of eligibility for relief (thus radically decreasing access to care), it also led to lesser pay for medical officers, as a competitive commercial tendering system guaranteed that positions went to the lowest bidder. This, along with accusations of harshness for following the strict guidelines, effectively lowered the social status of the poor law medical officer, and was seen to cast a shadow of degradation over the medical profession as a whole.[195]

The Provincial Medical and Surgical Association (the precursor to the British Medical Association) was founded in 1832 with the intention of improving 'the Medical Art' and upholding 'the dignity of the profession', which included pressing for improvement in appointments under the New Poor Law.[196] A large feature on the PMSA in *Berrow's Worcester Journal* in July 1838 insists that the medical profession must free itself 'from the contaminating, the corrupting taint of that spurious principle of Liberalism that would "grind the faces of the poor," and deny to the conscientious and humane Medical practitioner his fair reward'. The profession should rather be governed by the 'better feelings of the heart' and not by capitalist self-interest, and the journal turns to the recently published fifth edition of Warren's *Diary* as evidence of the moral privilege and duty of the medical practitioner, which according to their account, is so often not fully realised.[197]

The medical critique of liberal political economics, and of capitalism more broadly, became a substantial discourse in *Blackwood's*. Moir's poem depicting the morally rather than the commercially motivated medical man, 'Hippocrates to the Ambassadors of Artaxerxes', was reprinted in *Blackwood's* in 1836 during the vehement outcry against the New Poor Law of 1834 and the ongoing controversy over provision for the destitute in Scotland and Ireland. W. P.

Alison, in particular, turned to *Blackwood's* to forward what Christopher Hamlin deems his 'medical critique of industrialism and capitalism'.[198] The next chapter will examine how medical writers drew upon the ideological context of *Blackwood's* and also the *Quarterly Review* to develop and popularise their 'political medicine', and how this particular version of medical humanism was thus shaped and harnessed by conservative politics.

Notes

1. [Samuel Warren], 'Passages from the Diary of a Late Physician. Chap. I. Early Struggles', *BEM*, 28 (August 1830), 322–38 (p. 322).
2. Samuel Warren to William Blackwood, 24 February 1833, NLS MS 4037, fols 167–8.
3. Holloway, 'Medical Education in England', p. 324.
4. Standard accounts include Peterson, *The Medical Profession in Mid-Victorian London*, pp. 5–39, and Waddington, *The Medical Profession in the Industrial Revolution*, pp. 53–132.
5. Larson, *The Rise of Professionalism*, p. 24.
6. On 'quack' versus 'regular' medicine, see Bynum and Porter (eds), *Medical Fringe & Medical Orthodoxy*; Porter, *Quacks*.
7. Shortt, 'Physicians, Science, and Status'.
8. Worthington, *The Rise of the Detective*, p. 50.
9. Ibid. pp. 46–7.
10. Kennedy, 'The Ghost in the Clinic', p. 328.
11. Duncan, *Scott's Shadow*, p. 226.
12. See 'Introduction' to the *New Monthly Magazine*, 1821–54, in *The Wellesley Index to Victorian Periodicals*, available at http://wellesley.chadwyck.co.uk.ezproxy.lib.gla.ac.uk/toc/toc.do?id=JID-NMM&divLevel=1&action=new&queryId=#scroll (last accessed 18 September 2014).
13. Parker, *Literary Magazines and British Romanticism*, p. 141.
14. [Thomas Campbell], 'Preface', *NMM*, 1 (January 1821), iii–xii (p. v); See Sweet, 'The *New Monthly Magazine* and the Liberalism of the 1820s'.
15. Ibid. p. 149, p. 147.
16. Redding, *Fifty Years' Recollections*, vol. 2, p. 328.
17. [Warren], 'Early Struggles', p. 322.
18. Ibid. p. 322.
19. Ibid. p. 322.

20. 'The Guardian of Health. No. I. On the Character of Physicians', *NMM*, 1 (March 1814), 130–4 (p. 132).
21. Ibid. p. 132.
22. 'The Physician. No. I. On the Characteristics of Natural Health', *NMM*, 5 (September 1822), 254–8 (p. 254).
23. On medical patronage systems in the eighteenth century, see Jewson, 'Medical Knowledge and the Patronage System'.
24. [Thomas Richards], 'Professional Sketches. No. I. Mr. Abernethy', *NMM*, 23 (November 1828), 403–9 (p. 404).
25. Parker, *Literary Magazines and British Romanticism*, pp. 155–6.
26. [Thomas Richards], 'Professional Sketches. No. III. Dr. Armstrong and the College of Physicians', *NMM*, 25 (January 1829), 39–46 (p. 39).
27. Ibid. p. 43.
28. Ibid. p. 43.
29. Ibid. p. 44.
30. Ibid. p. 45.
31. 'Professional Puffs', *LMG*, 3 (28 February 1829), 422–6.
32. 'A Letter to the Yellow Goth, From the Author of "Professional Sketches," in the New Monthly Magazine, in reply to his Fulminating Article, in the Medical Mouthpiece of Messrs. Longman & Co.', *The Lancet*, 11 (14 March 1829), 760–2 (p. 761).
33. Porter and Porter, *Patient's Progress*, p. 119.
34. [Warren], 'Early Struggles', p. 331.
35. Ibid. p. 326.
36. Ibid. p. 333, p. 334.
37. Ibid. p. 334.
38. Ibid. p. 338.
39. Ibid. p. 326, p. 325.
40. Ibid. p. 327, p. 329.
41. [Samuel Warren?], 'The Young Surgeon. No. I', *NMM*, 25 (April 1829), 345–52 (p. 345).
42. [Samuel Warren?], 'The Young Surgeon. No. III', *NMM*, 26 (July 1829), 11–16 (p. 12).
43. [Wilson], 'Health and Longevity', p. 98.
44. [Wilson], 'Clark on Climate', p. 381.
45. [Warren], 'Early Struggles', p. 322.
46. Warren, 'Preface', in *Passages from the Diary of a Late Physician*, 5th edn, vol. 1, p. viii.
47. See C. R. B. Dunlop, 'Warren, Samuel (1807–1877)', in *ODNB*, available at http://www.oxforddnb.com/view/article/28792 (last accessed 20 June 2016) and 'Samuel Warren, Esq., Q.C., D.C.L. &c.', *The Illustrated Review*, 2.24 (2 October 1871), 193–5.

48. Samuel Warren to Alexander Blackwood, 22 October 1839, NLS MS 4049, fols 239–40.

49. William Blackwood to Samuel Warren, 25 December 1830, NLS MS 4732, fols 7–8.

50. William Blackwood to Samuel Warren, postmarked 23 February 1831, NLS MS 4732, fols 15–16.

51. 'Literary Criticism', *The Day, a Morning Journal of Literature, Fine Arts, Fashion &c.*, 74 (24 March 1832), 295; Samuel Warren, 'Introduction', in *Passages from the Diary of a Late Physician*, People's Edition, p. xii; William Blackwood to Samuel Warren, postmarked 25 August 1830, NLS MS 4732, fols 3–4; Samuel Warren to William Blackwood, 8 February 1831, MS 4031, fols 185–6.

52. Samuel Warren to Alexander Blackwood, 18 November 1835, NLS MS 4041, fols 263–4. Warren is referring to W. H. Harrison, *Tales of a Physician* (London: Robert Jennings, 1829).

53. 'Blackwood's Magazine v. the Secrets of the Medical Profession', *The Lancet*, 14 (28 August 1830), 878–9 (p. 879).

54. [Samuel Warren], 'Passages from the Diary of a late Physician. Chap. III. Note to the Editor – Intriguing and Madness – The Broken Heart', *BEM*, 28 (October 1830), 608–23 (p. 608).

55. 'The Physician's Diary, in Blackwood', *LMG*, 7 (23 October 1830), 118–19.

56. Samuel Warren to William Blackwood, 10 September 1830, NLS MS 4028, fols 300–1.

57. Samuel Warren to William Blackwood, 8 October 1830, NLS MS 4028, fols 303–4.

58. Samuel Warren to William Blackwood, 8 February 1831, NLS MS 4031, fols 185–6.

59. Samuel Warren to William Blackwood, 2 August 1832, NLS MS 4034, fols 268–9.

60. Robert Macnish to D. M. Moir, 22 October 1831, NLS Acc 9856, No. 49.

61. D. M. Moir to William Blackwood, September 1830, NLS MS 4028, fols 70–1.

62. D. M. Moir to William Blackwood, [end of October 1830], NLS MS 4028, fols 74–5.

63. [Moir], 'Why are Professional Men Indifferent Poets?', p. 41.

64. [Samuel Warren], 'Passages from the Diary of a Late Physician. Chap. II. Cancer; – The Dentist and the Comedian; – A Scholar's Death-Bed; – Preparing for the House ; – Duelling', *BEM*, 28 (September 1830, Part II), 474–86 (p. 474).

65. Ibid. p. 475.

66. Ibid. p. 475.
67. Ibid. p. 476.
68. Richardson, *Death, Dissection and the Destitute*, p. 31.
69. Robert Macnish to D. M. Moir, [January 1832?], NLS Acc. 9856, No. 50; see Robert Macnish to William Blackwood, 4, 24, and 27 February 1831, NLS MS 4030, fols 127–32.
70. [Samuel Warren], 'Passages from the Diary of a Late Physician. Chap. IV. Consumption – The Spectral Dog – The Forger', *BEM*, 28 (November 1830), 770–93 (p. 782).
71. Ibid. p. 782; on Reid and natural signs, see above, p. 12.
72. [Lockhart], *Peter's Letters*, vol. 1, p. 176; see above p. 88.
73. In my use of the term 'genre' here, I follow the parameters set by Class in 'Introduction: Medical Case Histories as Genre: New Approaches', pp. vii–xvi.
74. 'Preface, by the American Publishers', *Affecting Scenes*, vol. 1, p. iii.
75. Ibid. p. iv, p. v.
76. Miller, *Three Deaths and Enlightenment Thought*, p. 33.
77. 'Sir Herbert Taylor's Narrative of the Last Illness and Death of his Royal Highness the Duke of York', *BEM*, 21 (May 1827), 626–40 (p. 626).
78. Noble, 'John Wilson (Christopher North) and the Tory Hegemony', p. 146, p. 148.
79. Connell, *Romanticism, Economics, and the Question of 'Culture'*, p. 236, p. 237.
80. [J. G. Lockhart], 'The Family Library', *BEM*, 26 (September 1829), p. 416, as cited by Ibid. p. 237.
81. *Lives of British Physicians*, p. vii.
82. Warren, 'Preface to the Present Edition', in *Passages from the Diary of a Late Physician*, People's Edition, p. v.
83. [Warren], 'A Scholar's Death-Bed', p. 477.
84. Ibid. p. 480.
85. Ibid. p. 478.
86. Ibid. p. 486.
87. [Samuel Warren], 'Passages from the Diary of a Late Physician. Chap. XIV. The Magdalen', *BEM*, 32 (December 1832), 878–911 (p. 878).
88. On the philosophical background, see Tom L. Beauchamp, 'Common Sense and Virtue in the Scottish Moralists', in Baker, Porter, and Porter (eds), *The Codification of Medical Morality*, pp. 99–121.
89. Robert Baker, 'Introduction' to 'Part Two, The Eighteenth-Century Philosophical Background', in Baker, Porter, and Porter (eds), *The Codification of Medical Morality*, p. 94. Baker's quotations are from John Gregory, *Lectures on the Duties and Qualifications of*

a Physician (1772) as published in America by M. Carey & Son, Philadelphia, 1817, p. 22.

90. McCullough, *John Gregory and the Invention of Professional Medical Ethics*, p. 6; Haakonssen, *Medicine and Morals in the Enlightenment*, pp. 46–93.

91. John Gregory, *Lectures on the Duties and Qualifications of a Physician* (1772) in McCullough, *John Gregory's Writings on Medical Ethics*, pp. 162–245 (p. 166).

92. Ibid. pp. 166–7.

93. [Warren], 'A Scholar's Death-Bed', p. 483.

94. [Samuel Warren], 'Passages from the Diary of a Late Physician. Ch. XVI. The Merchant's Clerk', *BEM*, 40 (July 1836), 1–33 (p. 9).

95. [Samuel Warren], 'Passages from the Diary of a Late Physician. Ch. XVII. The Merchant's Clerk – Continued', *BEM*, 40 (August 1836), 181–207 (p. 185).

96. Charon, *Narrative Medicine*, p. 4.

97. Baker, 'Introduction' to 'Part Two, The Eighteenth-Century Philosophical Background', in Baker, Porter, and Porter (eds), *The Codification of Medical Morality*, pp. 93–8, (p. 94).

98. On the significance of Gregory, see ibid. pp. 93–8.

99. See Mary E. Fissell, 'Innocent and Honorable Bribes: Medical Manners in Eighteenth-Century Britain', in Baker, Porter, and Porter (eds), *The Codification of Medical Morality*, pp. 19–45.

100. Ibid. p. 32.

101. Ibid. p. 41.

102. Baker, 'Introduction' to 'Part Two, The Eighteenth-Century Philosophical Background', in Baker, Porter, and Porter (eds), *The Codification of Medical Morality*, p. 94.

103. See McCullough, *John Gregory and the Invention of Professional Medical Ethics*, pp. 95–6.

104. Warren, 'Preface to the Present Edition', in *Passages from the Diary of a Late Physician*, People's Edition, p. vi.

105. McCullough, *John Gregory and the Invention of Professional Medical Ethics*, p. 219.

106. Ibid. p. 232.

107. Ibid. p. 266.

108. [Samuel Warren], 'Passages from the Diary of a Late Physician. Chap. V. A "Man About Town". – Death at the Toilet', *BEM*, 28 (December 1830), 921–40 (p. 932).

109. Ibid. p. 933.

110. Exemplary texts include: Percival, *Medical Ethics*; 'A Lecture on the Conduct and Duties of the Medical Practitioner, Delivered at

the Theatre, Great Windmill Street, Oct. 5, By B. C. Brodie, F.R.S.',
LMG, 5 (10 October 1829), 39–45; Abercrombie, *Inquiries Concerning the Intellectual Powers*; Halford, *On the Education and Conduct
of a Physician*; Brodie, 'Introductory Discourse', in *The Works of Sir
Benjamin Collins Brodie*, vol. 1, pp. 485–505.

111. [Warren], 'A "Man About Town"', p. 924.
112. Ibid. p. 924.
113. Ibid. p. 932.
114. Gregory, *Lectures on the Duties and Qualifications of a Physician*
     (1772), in McCullough, *John Gregory's Writings on Medical Ethics
     and Philosophy of Medicine*, p. 187.
115. [Warren], 'A "Man About Town"', p. 936.
116. Ibid. p. 924.
117. Percival, *Medical Ethics*, p. 192.
118. Ibid. p. 193.
119. Abercrombie, *Inquiries Concerning the Intellectual Powers*, p. 431.
120. Ibid. p. 423.
121. Abercrombie, *Inquiries Concerning the Intellectual Powers*, 11th edn,
     p. 454.
122. [Samuel Warren], 'Passages from the Diary of a Late Physician.
     Chap. IV. Consumption – The Spectral Dog – The Forger', *BEM*, 28
     (November 1830), p. 788.
123. Ibid. p. 788.
124. Ibid. p. 792, p. 793.
125. Kennedy, 'The Ghost in the Clinic', p. 330.
126. [Warren], 'The Spectre-Smitten', p. 361.
127. [Samuel Warren], 'Passages from the Diary of a Late Physician. Chap.
     VI. The Turned Head – The Wife', *BEM*, 29 (January 1831), 105–27
     (p. 113).
128. Brody, *Stories of Sickness*, pp. 269–70.
129. [Samuel Warren], 'Passages from the Diary of a Late Physician. Ch.
     XI. The Ruined Merchant', *BEM*, 30 (July 1831), 60–82 (p. 60).
130. Ibid. pp. 60–1.
131. [Warren], 'The Spectre-Smitten', p. 371.
132. [Warren], *Passages from the Diary of a Late Physician* (1832), vol. 2,
     p. 17.
133. Charon, *Narrative Medicine*, p. vii.
134. Halford, *On the Deaths of Some Eminent Persons of Modern Times*,
     p. 40.
135. Samuel Warren to Alexander Blackwood, 21 February 1835, NLS MS
     4041, fols 248–9.
136. 'The Physician's Diary, in Blackwood', p. 119.

137. [Warren], 'Intriguing and Madness', p. 616.
138. 'College of Physicians. Monday, 1 June. *Observations on Insanity*. By Sir H. Halford', *LMG*, 4 (6 June 1829), 26–7; [Warren], 'Intriguing and Madness', p. 616.
139. For Halford's valuation of a classical education, see Halford, *On the Education and Conduct of a Physician*, pp. 7–10; and, for an example of the utility he saw in the study of 'the great poets of antiquity', see *Essays and Orations, Read and Delivered at the Royal College of Physicians*, p. 64.
140. As cited in G. T. Bettany (rev. Michael Bevan), 'Halford, Sir Henry, first baronet (1766–1844)', in *ODNB*, available at http://www.oxforddnb.com/view/article/11919 (last accessed 20 June 2016).
141. Halford, *On the Education and Conduct of a Physician*, p. 15, p. 17.
142. See McCullough, *John Gregory and the Invention of Professional Medical Ethics*, p. 218.
143. See Bettany, 'Halford, Sir Henry, first baronet (1766–1844)', in *ODNB*.
144. 'Some Passages from the Diary of Late Fashionable Apothecary', *NMM*, 31 (January 1831), 233–41 (p. 233).
145. Examples of this include: Adams, *Sketches from Life*, p. viii; Douglas, *Adventures of a Medical Student*, vol. 1, p. 11; *Extracts from the Diary of a Living Physician*, pp. iii–iv; [Rymer], *Manuscripts from the Diary of a Physician*, vol. 1, p. 3.
146. 'Some Passages from the Diary of Late Fashionable Apothecary', p. 233.
147. Ibid. p. 233.
148. Ibid. p. 238.
149. For an overview of the magazine and its politics, see Thrall, *Rebellious Fraser's*.
150. [William Maginn], 'Our "Confession of Faith."', *FM*, 1 (February 1830), 1–7 (p. 5). For a concise overview of the founding of *Fraser's*, see the 'Introduction' to *Fraser's* in *The Wellesley Index to Victorian Periodicals, 1824–1900*, available at http://wellesley.chadwyck.co.uk.ezproxy.lib.gla.ac.uk/toc/toc.do?id=JID-FM&divLevel=1&action=new&queryId=#scroll (last accessed 8 December 2015).
151. 'Introduction' to *Fraser's* in *The Wellesley Index to Victorian Periodicals*.
152. 'A Plea for Physicians', *FM*, 37 (March 1848), 286–94.
153. 'Introduction' to *Fraser's* in *The Wellesley Index to Victorian Periodicals*.
154. Fisher counts at least '38 articles and reviews in *Fraser's* between 1830 and 1838' which 'discussed, incidentally or centrally, the state of British letters, bewailing both the mediocrity of artistic work and the poverty of public taste' ('"In the Present Famine of Anything Substantial"', p. 108).

155. 'Notices to Correspondents', *FM*, 2 (August 1830), p. 8.

156. On defining quackery, see Porter, *Quacks*, pp. 11–13.

157. See for example [William Maginn and John Abraham Heraud], 'Mr. Edward Lytton Bulwer's [sic] Novels; and Remarks on Novel-Writing', *FM*, 5 (June 1830), 509–32.

158. [William Maginn], 'The Dominie's Legacy', *FM*, 1 (April 1830), 318–35 (p. 320), as quoted in Mason, '"The Quack Has Become God"', p. 14.

159. [J. A. Carlyle], 'On Medical Quackery and Mr. St. John Long', *FM*, 1 (May 1830), 451–6 (p. 452).

160. On Long, see Marten Hutt, 'Long, St John Long (1798–1834)', in *ODNB*, available at http://www.oxforddnb.com/view/article/16971 (last accessed 20 June 2016); [J. A. Carlyle], 'Medical Quackery and Mr. John St. John Long. No. II', *FM*, 2 (October 1830), 264–5; [William Maginn?], 'Visit from Mr John Saint Long', *FM*, 3 (April 1831), 365–8.

161. On *Fraser's* development of critical standards, see Newman, '"Prosecuting the Onus Criminus"'.

162. 'Notices to Correspondents', p. 8.

163. On continued popularity of the series, see D. M. Moir to William Blackwood, 2 January 1830 [corrected as 1831], NLS MS 4030, fols 189–90.

164. [J. A. Carlyle], 'Some Passages from the Diary of the late Mr. St. John Long', *FM*, 2 (January 1831), 739–40 (p. 739).

165. Ibid. p. 740.

166. 'Notices to Correspondents', p. 8.

167. Samuel Warren to William Blackwood, 8 December 1830, NLS MS 4028, fols 309–10.

168. Samuel Warren to William Blackwood, 18 November 1830, NLS MS 4028, fols 307–8; Samuel Warren to William Blackwood, 31 December 1830, NLS MS 4028, fols 311–12.

169. Leary, '*Fraser's Magazine* and the Literary Life', p. 109.

170. [William Maginn?], 'Regina and her Correspondents', *FM*, 6 (September 1832), 255–6 (p. 255).

171. 'The Real Diary of a Physician', *The Doctor, A Medical Magazine*, 1 (3 April 1833), 324.

172. Ibid. p. 324.

173. Johnson, *The Lives of the Poets*, vol. 2, p. 507.

174. See 'Remarkable Career. A. M. Adams Primus' Ancestry'; Adams, *A Dynasty of Doctors*; Webb, *Wish You Were Here*.

175. Adams, *Sketches from Life*, p. viii.

176. Ibid. p. 2.

177. Ibid. p. 20, p. 5.

178. Ibid. p. 62.

179. Ibid. p. 69.

180. Ibid. p. 72.

181. Ibid. p. 74.

182. Ibid. p. 74.

183. Ibid. p. 74.

184. Ibid. pp. 190–1.

185. Ibid. p. 191.

186. Ibid. p. vii.

187. Ibid. p. viii.

188. 'Experiences of a Surgeon. No. IV. – A Dissecting-Room Incident', *MM*, 1 (June 1835), 567–75 (p. 570).

189. For references to the stethoscope, see [Anthony Todd Thomson], 'Sketches from the Note-book of a Physician. – No. V. On the Nature, the Causes, and the Prevention of Consumption', *NMM*, 59 (June 1840), 227–39 (p. 238); [Anthony Todd Thomson], 'Sketches from the Note-book of a Physician. No. VI. On the Prevention of Consumption', *NMM*, 59 (August 1840), 506–16 (p. 512).

190. [Robert Douglas], 'Reminiscences of a Medical Student. No. XII. An Excursion with Bob Whyte', *NMM*, 67 (March 1843), 392–410 (p. 392).

191. *Extracts from the Diary of a Living Physician*, edited by L.F.C. (1851), also follows this general pattern. The text is equally moralistic but, while portraying dramatic cases and a physician's benevolent acts, focuses rather on clinical decisions and actions rather than emotive responses; however, I have been unable to verify if it was written by a medical practitioner or is a Warren-like hoax. An example of this recalibration (that falls outwith the date range of this book) is Dr John Staples' *The Diary of a London Physician* (1863). An interesting exception to this trend is Dr J. Slade's *Alice Glynn: A Tale, From the Diary of a Physician* (1845). In the opening, the narrator declares: 'I, less than most men, could look coolly on the scenes and occurrences daily practice brought before me. Many a times I have bit my lip to hide its trembling, or closed my eye to conceal the tear that trickled to it.' However, unlike the general claims to verisimilitude within this genre, in the 'Advertisement' Slade explains his intention to formulate the tale as a 'lengthened romance'.

192. Brown, 'Rab and his Friends', in *Horæ Subsecivæ*, p. 305.

193. Ibid. p. 305, p. 307.

194. Hamlin, *Public Health and Social Justice*, p. 93.

195. See Loudon, *Medical Care and the General Practitioner*, pp. 228–48.

196. 'Supplement' to the *Berrow's Worcester Journal* (26 July 1838). I. 7078. On the PMSA and poor law reform, see Hamlin, *Public Health and Social Justice*, pp. 93–4; on the founding of the PMSA, see Parry and Parry, *The Rise of the Medical Profession*, p. 126; P. W. J. Bartrip, 'Hastings, Sir Charles (1794–1866)', in *ODNB*, available at http://www.oxforddnb.com/view/article/12560?docPos=9 (last accessed 20 June 2016).
197. The citation of Warren may be found in *Berrow's Worcester Journal* (26 July 1838), I. 7078, while my quotation is from the 'Supplement' to the *Berrow's Worcester Journal* (26 July 1838), I. 7078.
198. Hamlin, *Public Health and Social Justice*, p. 81.

Chapter 5

The Rise of Public Health in the Popular Periodical Press: The Political Medicine of W. P. Alison, Robert Gooch, and Robert Ferguson

"Poor Simon's sick." "Then for the Doctor send."
  "The Union Doctor? He lives far away –
  Seven miles, and has seven parishes, they say,
And his own private practice to attend.
Besides, sick Simon has no idle friend,
  Where all must work; nor has he pence to pay;
Nor comes the Doctor without order penn'd
  By th' Overseer – and this is market-day."[1]

As David Hamilton has noted, '[i]t was in the pages of the *Edinburgh Review* and *Blackwoods* [sic] *Magazine* that the first signs of the growth of power of central government in health matters can be seen'.[2] Hamilton is referring to the vehement debates regarding poor law reform that featured in both periodicals in the 1830s and 1840s. In *Blackwood's* the debate was pursued across factual articles, fiction and even poetry. For example, the above quoted sonnet on 'Parish Sick and Parish Doctor', published in *Blackwood's* in April 1838, criticises the system of medical provision for the poor in England following the New Poor Law of 1834 as officious, ineffective, and controlled by the commercial forces represented by the 'market-day'. While the rise of public health is most often associated with sanitary reform and the work of Edwin Chadwick (1800–90), prior to the shift towards eradicating filth proselytised by Chadwick's *Report on the Sanitary Condition of the Labouring Population of Great Britain* (1842), commentators on public health focused on social rather than environmental issues. They were concerned with the question of how far the central government should intercede in alleviating the miseries of poverty and the poor working conditions associated with industrial labour.[3] The burgeoning field thus became a major site for the ideological clash between liberals devoted to Malthusian political economics (and thus minimal state intervention) and progressive Tories who instead argued for a paternalistic and often morally and religiously oriented approach. Given their political alignments, it is unsurprising that *Blackwood's* and the *Edinburgh Review* often served as platforms for these opposing points of view.[4]

Hamlin recounts how in the early nineteenth century,

> [a]n age of benevolence, rooted in the elevation of sentiment and the presumption of a 'moral economy' regulating social relations, gives way to an age of austere political economy, thriving on conflict and rooted in what are conceived the natural laws of human society, like those espoused by Ebenezer Scrooge.[5]

Two *Blackwood's* contributors who are the focus of this chapter, W. P. Alison and Robert Gooch, contributed to the development of a Romantic medical counter-discourse – a humanistic 'political medicine' (a term I borrow from Hamlin) that critiqued liberal political economists and utilitarianism and promoted the importance of moral feelings and Christian sentiments in informing public health policy. These two figures occupy distinct political epochs and are concerned with different geographical locales; both, however, subscribe to the essential Blackwoodian vision of 'paternalism' – 'a mind that infused political theory with religious faith; that trusted to order, tradition, and experience more than to agitation, innovation and abstract reasoning', and which pleaded for 'organic communities tied together by personal bonds' in stark contrast to 'the utilitarians and their world of calculating individuals'.[6] By way of contrast, I shall turn to Robert Ferguson, the key medical contributor to the *Quarterly Review* from 1829 to 1854. Although Ferguson also contributed to what David Roberts terms 'the social conscience of Tory periodicals', writing on issues relevant to public health and promoting a paternalistic approach, his writings more clearly reflect the counter-revolutionary agenda of the *Quarterly*, as opposed to the more explicit humanism of *Blackwood's*.[7]

W. P. Alison and the Poor Law Debate

In an article for *Blackwood's* on 'The Factory System' in April 1833, written in support of a Ten Hour Bill, John Wilson contrasts the perceived methodology of the political economists with that of medical men, to the disadvantage of the former. The political economists 'HAVE NO FACTS' yet 'theorize without them, and out of two or three puny observations, proceed, by way of induction, to establish general laws'.[8] While mocking certain medical practitioners who acted as witnesses against the proposed Cotton Mills and Factories Act in 1818 as 'audacious blockheads' for insisting that they 'HAVE NO FACTS' to affirm that factory work is unhealthy, Wilson applauds the work of other medical men whose testimony, based on 'observation and practice', as well as an ability to make judgements derived from their 'knowledge of the nature of things', asserts the importance of the 'Vital Economy' over 'Political Economy'.[9] Interestingly, in Wilson's article, a 'good doctor' narrative lies at the heart of his critique of political economy, with his detailed praise of certain medical men examined before the Committees of 1818 and 1832 standing in stark juxtaposition to his critique of the flawed theorising and 'hardened' hearts of the political economists.[10]

The following month, in May 1833, in his article 'On Poor's Laws, and their Introduction into Ireland', Wilson explicitly states the role that he believes the medical profession (rather than the political economists) should play in advising legislative change: 'medical, which in this case is moral, science, must study the causes of health and disease; and the antidotes and remedies which are thus discovered, it is the duty of the state to apply'.[11] However, despite such affirmations of medical authority, the medical profession never remains long unscathed in *Blackwood's*. The contemporaneous critique and celebration of two opposing types of medical professionals in 'The Factory System' is characteristic, and through the 1820s and 1830s, 'bad doctor' narratives also contribute to the magazine's critique of political economy. A Swiftian satire published in 1822 by J. G. Lockhart, which uses the logic of political economy to propose that all persons be dissected post-mortem and their bodies then turned into useful objects, is echoed by John Eagles in 'New Scheme for Maintaining the Poor' in April 1838, where he proposes a similarly extreme utilitarian regime (also akin to that proposed in Henry Thomson's satire,

'Panaceas for Poverty', in December 1823) while decrying medical provision in England under the New Poor Law.[12] The previous year, Eagles's article 'Medical Attendance and Other Parochials' explains how, under the New Poor Law, the 'poor are farmed out at a few far-things per head – a price at which none but the lowest of the profes-sion can come forward, or those upon the advantage thereby offered of *subjects* for experiment'.[13] Given the associations between disease, destitution, and dissection (to borrow Ruth Richardson's alliteration) solidified in the Anatomy Act of 1832, such statements are unsurpris-ing. These articles evoke a nightmarish world in which the 'march of intellect' prevails at the cost of natural feeling: political economy replaces moral economy.

This was the context in which Alison published two key articles – 'Evils of the State of Ireland' and 'Justice to Ireland – a Poor Law', in October and December 1836 respectively – which would form the intellectual core of his most important contribution to the poor law debate, *Observations on the Management of the Poor in Scotland, and its Effects on the Health of Great Towns* (1840), considered to be 'one of the most influential pamphlets published in early Victorian Scotland'.[14] Alison argued that, while Malthus's general principal of population was correct, his deduction that the monetary assistance provided by poor laws only perpetuates poverty by discouraging 'moral restraint' and thus encouraging population growth did not hold up to experience.[15] Rather, Alison argued, the 'tendency (inher-ent in human nature) to outstrip the means of subsistence, is most effectively restrained where a fixed and uniform provision, securing [the poor] against destitution and degradation, is known to exist'.[16] While Thomas Chalmers preached the importance of religious and moral instruction in promoting moral restraint, drawing upon his practical experience among the poor in Edinburgh, Alison believed that destitution and degradation incapacitated human beings from making rational decisions that might prevent future misery and thus future susceptibility to disease, since '[a] certain degree of physical comfort is essential to the permanent development, and the habitual influence over human conduct, of any feelings higher than our sen-sual appetites'.[17] Education was futile until certain basic needs were met, and the Scottish system that provided no systematic relief for the able-bodied, beyond charitable offerings managed by the kirk, was insufficient. Alison maintained that providential design, natural feelings and biblical teachings affirmed his argument: '[t]he relief of human suffering is a sacred duty, written from the beginning on the hearts of men, enforced by the positive precepts of the Gospel, and which no nation can violate or neglect with impunity'.[18] The posited causal connection between destitution and contagious fever, the medical core of Alison's argument, meant that violation or neglect of these duties would be the gateway to epidemic disease.[19]

'Evils of the State of Ireland' opens with a Burkean appeal to the 'feeling' of the 'true Conservative', who must find the 'human suffering' in Ireland a 'perpetual source of horror and humiliation'. Referring to those who promote '[t]he idea, that all regular systematic relief given to the poor only encourages improvidence, fosters population, and ultimately increases poverty', Alison laments that 'we find it pretty generally doubted by such reasoners in our own country, whether any men can have strong heads, who suffer their hearts to be touched by the sight of want and misery'.[20] Wilson had already linked Scottish intellectual opposition to poor laws with the national blight long lamented by *Blackwood's*, declaring 'We are a worthy, and a rational, and no [sic] very immoral or irreligious race, but we have a better right to pride ourselves on our prudence than our benevolence, and the whole nation doth too often look like a School of Utilitarians.'[21] This intellectual opposition was propagated at this time in the *Edinburgh Review*, which supported the stricter provisions of the New Poor Law while opposing both the introduction of a poor law in Ireland and the reformation of the Scottish poor law.[22] Malthus's doctrines were attacked in *Blackwood's*, despite attempts by *Edinburgh Review* contributors such as Henry Reeve to refute the charge that they stifle '"the finer feelings of the heart"'.[23] Thus, Alison is able to appeal to the supposed division between intellect and feeling that underlay the Romantic ideology of *Blackwood's* and to present his political medicine as a recuperative intervention justified by both 'facts and reasonings' and 'the natural feelings of humanity'.[24]

For Wilson, perhaps unsurprisingly, poetry is the answer. In 'The Factory System', he laments the 'hardened' hearts of the political economists and presents the 'sacred genius of William Wordsworth' – in whose works 'Poetry, and Moral Philosophy, and Christianity, and Political Economy' are 'all in one' – as a corrective to 'the dicta that drivel in dust from the cold hard lips of an oracle of dry bones, such as Peter Macculloch'.[25] The poetry of Ebenezer Elliot (1781–1849), 'the greatest Poet of the Poor', is cited as 'impassioned truth' – as fact combined with feeling.[26] Alison also turns to '[p]oetry and eloquence'[27] in 'Justice to Ireland', where he cites 'the words of [Walter Scott's] Meg Merrilies' to express the feelings of ejected tenants and thus to explain why they often become lawless and shed the moral restraint required to stem excess population growth.[28] Alison's literary appeal functions together with his call 'to enter the houses' of the destitute to better understand the need for an effective poor law. As Hamlin has observed, Alison's social medicine, a union of the philosophical and environmentalist traditions of Stewart and Cullen, was informed by 'the imagined subjectivity of persons in particular social situations'.[29]

In this, Alison's contributions resonate with Warren's *Passages from the Diary of a Late Physician*, the fictional representation, as outlined in the previous chapter, of a physician who must 'enter the houses' of the diseased and destitute.[30] Although it was thought to cater to the tastes of the well-to-do, a link between poverty and disease pervades Warren's series, from the 'Early Struggles' of the late physician's own young family to cases such as 'The Merchant's Clerk', published in July and August 1836, just two months before Alison's first contribution to *Blackwood's* on the poor law debate. While Warren does not address poor law reform directly, some contemporaries clearly saw the relevance of his series to the debate. In July 1831, an advertisement appeared in the *Liverpool Mercury* under the header '*Miseries of the Irish*', announcing:

> Amongst the contents of the next *Kaleidoscope*, will be found a notice of a heart-rending picture of domestic wretchedness, such as is now experienced by thousands of our miserable and famishing fellow-creatures in Ireland. It is from one of the papers in *Blackwood*, entitled, 'Passages from the Diary of a Late Physician.' Although the narrative is in all probability a work of fiction, the best authenticated accounts from Ireland prove that scenes even more appalling than any work of imagination has ever portrayed, are now matters of daily and hourly occurrence in that ill-fated country.[31]

The advertisement mistakenly locates the case of the O'Hurdle family, related in Warren's 'Rich and Poor' in June 1831, in Ireland rather than in London, but in doing so brings the case into dialogue

with the campaign for an Irish poor law. The *Kaleidoscope* makes
no such mistake and rather emphasises the plight of the urban poor
more broadly, giving their extract from Warren's 'affecting narrative'
the title 'To What Miseries are not the Poor Exposed?' and prefacing
it with an expression of the desire 'to awaken the unthinking and
the opulent to a sense of the calamitous condition of the *poverty
stricken* people'.[32] In an anti-Malthusian rhetorical gesture, the preface depicts poverty and its associated miseries not as punishments
for imprudence but as afflictions to which 'our destitute fellow-sub-
jects are the devoted prey'. The extract represents the extreme misery
of the O'Hurdle family, housed together in a wretched garret, as the
result of a cascading series of calamities. The husband is asthmatic
and unable to work; the wife has just given birth and now has yet
another starving child; and both have starved themselves and their
children to hire an attorney to defend their eldest son against a false
accusation of robbery.[33] Their story is related by the wife and mother
herself. When the late physician asks, 'How many of you are ill?' she
answers: 'we all of us are! Ah, your honour! – A 'Firmary, without
physic or victuals!' The link between destitution and disease is made
abundantly clear, as is the insufficiency of the 'paltry pittance from
the parish' to ameliorate it.[34]

Hamlin has highlighted how Chadwick's *Sanitary Report* of July
1842, rarely including a 'subject's eye view', systematically worked
to 'invalidate the subjectivity of those who lived in overcrowded
dwellings or poorly built cottages'.[35] He also notes that Alison, in
contrast to Chadwick and the other medical men who contributed
to the *Local Reports for Scotland* (1842), was unique in not viewing
the poor as 'an alien and dangerous population'. He asserted, on the
contrary, that '[t]o appreciate how people might act to check population one had to gauge how they viewed their own lives – what they
hoped for, what they thought they could control, how they made
choices'.[36] In short, Alison's methodology, emphasising the need to
understand the actual conditions of poverty and to value the subjective experience of the suffering poor, is not unlike that of Warren's
late physician, who seeks sympathetic engagement with the narratives of even his most deprived patients.[37] While lacking the Gothic
sensationalism of Warren's series, Alison's writings on public health
appeal to a similar humanistic ethos.

It is well known that literary texts, and particularly those published in the popular periodical press, played a dynamic role as the 'popular front' of the debates surrounding poor law reform and the 'condition of England' question.[38] What I wish to emphasise is that Alison – the most important contributor to the campaign for a Scottish poor law – chose to first present his arguments to the public in the pages of a literary magazine that provided an ideological framing for his humanistic approach, both through discursive articles, such as those by Wilson, and through its more 'literary' contents. When Alison writes, in October 1836, that '[t]he wealth of a nation is not the result of a mere process of arithmetic. It is the work of human hands, and is guided by the impulse of human feelings', he draws upon the Romantic ideology of *Blackwood's* to forward his humanistic political medicine.[39] Alison was not the first medical contributor to do this. In the next section, I introduce the work of Robert Gooch, whose contributions to *Blackwood's* preceded Alison's articles on the condition of Ireland, and likewise use the Blackwoodian context to forward a progressive Tory social medicine.

Robert Gooch and the Making of a Progressive Tory Social Medicine

Robert Gooch was highly regarded for the clarity of his thinking and writing as well as for his utilisation of apt and vivid illustrations.[40] In a period when specialised medical writing was increasingly seen as inappropriate for publication in general periodicals, Gooch was particularly adept at harnessing the polemical power of the popular press to forward his political medicine. As Jonathan Cutmore notes in his study of the *Quarterly Review*, Gooch's 1825 article on 'Plague, a Contagious Disease', arguing against a proposed appeal of the quarantine laws published in the Benthamite *Westminster Review*, was heralded by some as 'the first article in the journal's history that demonstrably had an impact on legislation'.[41] Richardson cites Gooch's review of 'A Bill for Preventing the Disinterment of Human Bodies, and for Regulating Schools of Anatomy', published in the *Quarterly* in January 1830, as a significant contribution to the public debate leading up to the Anatomy Act of 1832.[42] In a letter to

John Murray accompanying his 'short article on the Anatomy Bill', Gooch notes:

> As the subject will be discussed early in the next session of Parliament it should be put in a the Xmas number that is if Lockhart should approve of it – I have directed my fire not a [sic] medical men but at the Public and our Legislation so that there is not a word or a thought which is not suited to the general Reader.[43]

From April 1826 Gooch held the position of librarian to the king, a post that provided financial security during the prolonged illness that led to his early death in 1830.[44] In a subsequent letter to Murray he requests a separate copy of his article to show to his Majesty. A bound 'red morocco one', kindly supplied by Murray, was deemed 'worthy of its destination'.[45]

The position was a notable achievement for a man born to a family of limited circumstances. However, Gooch was highly industrious and also had a talent for making advantageous friendships. While his family could not afford to provide him with a classical education, he taught himself Greek and Latin, and during his apprenticeship to a surgeon apothecary in Yarmouth, Norfolk, he befriended a blind gentleman, a Mr Harley, whom he read to in his leisure hours. In return, Harley 'helped him develop a taste for history, literature, chemistry, and philosophy, which remained with him for the rest of his life'.[46] When Gooch matriculated at Edinburgh, he was a suitable companion for Henry Herbert Southey (1783–1865), Robert Southey's younger brother, and William Knighton (1776–1836), later first baronet, who helped him to establish his London medical practice. This practice included the post of physician to the Westminster Lying-in Hospital and a lectureship in midwifery at St Bartholomew's Hospital. Knighton also facilitated his later intimacy with the royal household, but it was his relationship with Henry Southey that brought about his entrance onto the literary stage.[47]

Southey introduced Gooch to his brother, Robert, in the autumn of 1805, and, according to his posthumous life of Gooch in *Lives of British Physicians* (1830), the poet 'had liked him at first sight'.[48] By February 1812, Robert Southey was preparing the way for Gooch to become a fellow contributor to *Quarterly*, writing to Murray that 'Gooch is a very able man, – one of the most promising xxx of my friends; – & capable of being a useful assistant in the Quarterly. No man is more likely to distinguish himself in literature as well as in his own profession.'[49] In a follow-up letter of 1813, he notes that 'His mind is clear & comprehensive, his style animated & perspicuous, & his taste has that intuition [which is] never to be found except where the moral sense is as carefully cultivated as the intellect.'[50] However, Gooch would not publish his first contribution to the *Quarterly* until April 1822.[51]

While his desire to contribute to the periodical press was clearly driven by the need to supplement his income, by 1825 Gooch was sufficiently socially connected to be seen as a potential asset to publishers. He was first introduced as a potential contributor to *Blackwood's* by his younger friend and protegé Robert Ferguson, who in his letter of introduction explains that he is sending a '"Month's Tour" in France' by Gooch, 'a man, high in the profession', which he believes 'will not suit' Blackwood. However, he advises 'it would be worth your while to secure him if possible ~~by~~ for his connection among the nobility is so extensive & his xxx habits so intimate that of course his friends would read his articles and thus increase the sale of your xxx <u>already all-pervading Magazine</u>'.[52] While a 'Month's Tour' was not ultimately accepted, an account of 'Two Days with Dr. Parr' appeared in November 1825. Gooch followed up with some short pieces to go under the header of 'Blackwoodiana', and reported that he was writing a review of another novel by Christoph Martin Wieland (to follow a recent review by Ferguson). In the next few months he submitted two medical articles, 'Protestant Sisters of Charity' and 'The Quarterly Review of Dr Marmichael on Contagion and the Plague'.[53]

In 'Two Days with Dr. Parr', Gooch indulges his love of anecdote, or 'Goochiana's' as Southey termed it, in an account of two memorable encounters with the late classicist Samuel Parr (1747–1825).[54] He relates how he and a group of friends tracked Parr down in Warwick, where they heard he was attending a meeting of a Bible Society. Over a convivial dinner Parr declared that the 'most desirable' profession

> for a man of intellect was that of physic; the practice of the law, he said, spoiled a man's moral sense and philosophic spirit; the Church was too bigoted and stiff-starched; the study and practice of physic was equally favourable to a man's moral sentiments and intellectual faculties.[55]

Gooch appears to agree with Parr, in part at least, so long as the motivation for practising physic is grounded in Christian devotion. The following month Gooch promotes a scheme to improve the provision of medical care to the country poor by forming a religious order of nurses, the 'Protestant Sisters of Charity'. In outlining the need for such an order he delineates the three primary motivations for those currently charged with caring for the sick: 'scientific zeal', 'natural humanity', and, lastly, 'mercenary motives'.[56] All these he declares,

> cannot be trusted to for steady attention – the one subsides with the solution of a question, the other hardens by habit, the last requires jealous inspection – there are long intervals of indifference, and apathy, and inattention – we want an actuating motive of a more steady and enduring nature, which requires neither curiosity, nor emotion, nor avarice to keep it alive, which still burns in the most tranquil states of mind, and out of the reach of human inspection, and this motive is religion.[57]

Here Gooch applies the 'Edinburgh ideal of the good physician', motivated by a morality rooted in natural feeling and sustained through Christian duty, to his prospective order of female nurses. It was an ethical ideal that Gooch himself reflected in his public persona.[58]

Henry Southey's life of Gooch emphasises his religious devotion and benevolence, a theme further developed when a revised version of Gooch's life was included in the Religious Tract Society's *Sketches of Eminent Medical Men*. The autobiographical sketch inserted in 'Protestant Sisters of Charity' prepared the way for these readings of his life. Gooch relates an anecdote from his student days in which, while holidaying in Yarmouth during summer break in 1806, he was entrusted with the care of a wounded Frenchmen named Pierre, who was one of a large group brought onshore and housed in a temporary hospital after the English navy captured a French frigate. Gooch's anecdote draws upon the literary aesthetics of *Blackwood's*, featuring a pious and sentimentalised deathbed scene in the magazine's proto-Kailyard mode, whilst at the same time carefully documenting the progress of the medical case. Gooch vividly describes the amputation of Pierre's wounded leg and the pains he took to prevent what remained of his patient's limb from ulcerating due to extended bed rest. When he temporarily leaves his charge in the care of 'a young man, an assistant surgeon, who, although good tempered, and not deficient in sense or in knowledge of his profession, was incorrigibly indolent and inattentive', the wound ulcerates and leads to a fatal 'hectic fever'.[59] Gooch returns to the hospital to find Pierre in this unhappy plight, and the anecdote culminates with a tearful scene: Pierre dies happy that he is able to see his dutiful carer one last time. Gooch proceeds to appeal to 'that class of Christians in whom, above all others, religion is not a mere Sunday ceremony' to pour their religious enthusiasm into forming a new class of public caregivers who might prevent such needless tragedy.[60] In a letter to Blackwood, Moir complained that the piece 'smells a vast deal too much of the Shop, and though a neat enough little paper, propounds qua physician, a scheme that in medical practice would be found romantically ridiculous'.[61]

Gooch's 'Protestant Sisters of Charity', modelled on the Sœurs de la Charité, or Sisters of Charity, in Catholic countries, were to receive a 'practical medical education', and, more importantly, were also to manifest a quality of care sustained by religious piety.[62] Gooch's medical article contributes to the common agenda that linked the scientific articles in the early number of *Blackwood's*, their contribution to the magazine's steadfast opposition to the separation between science and religion, as well as to its persistent Romantic Tory demonisation of the commercial spirit.[63] In two articles he subsequently contributed to the *London Medical Gazette* under the couthy (and, at this point in his career, inaccurate) pseudonym 'A Country Surgeon', Gooch furthered his plea, describing the history of the Sisters of Charity in France and also presenting the Béguines, whose work and devotions he had witnessed first-hand in Bruges and Ghent, as a possible model for his order of 'religious female physicians'.[64] By way of juxtaposition, in his first article Gooch criticises the mercenary motivation of parish surgeons under the English Poor Law. According to Gooch, the parish overseers hired surgeons at the cheapest rate, whose position then enabled them to attract more wealthy patients, who distracted them from their duties to the poor. Gooch's description of the 'Rural Esculapius' who 'mounts his nag, envelops his throat in a handkerchief, buttons his fear-nought close about his chin, and, wrapping its skirts about his knees', rides many miles 'through sleet and snow, along road and lane, and hill and common', is not unlike Ian Maclaren's later *A Doctor of the Old*

School (1895). Instead of celebrating the dedicated country surgeon, however, Gooch's description emphasises the avarice which 'induces him to accept these degrading terms'.[65] It appears that the commercial dynamic deprecated in 'Parish Sick and Parish Doctor' was not unique to medical provision under the New Poor Law.

Gooch's work held common cause with Southey's progressive Tory politics and is indicative of the relationship between the humanistic medical culture promoted in *Blackwood's* and 'Romantic conservatism' more broadly. In his *Colloquies on the Progress and Prospects of Society* (1829), a series of dialogues between 'Montesinos' and 'Sir Thomas More' comparing pre-Reformation England with the present day, Southey includes both 'Protestant Sisters of Charity' and Gooch's articles in the *London Medical Gazette* as the sole appendices. The *Colloquies*, along with Coleridge's *On the Constitution of Church and State* (1830), is one of the key texts of Romantic conservativism, but, as David Eastwood has noted, the 'Romantic Conservatives' were not simply supporters of the Protestant constitutional orthodoxy. They were rather distinguished from 'more conventional, High Tories' by their 'faith in the positive possibilities of paternalistic state invention'.[66] In the *Colloquies*, for example, More at one point critiques the lack of a 'medical police' in the present day, blaming 'the notions of liberty in England' for allowing 'evils of every kind, physical, moral, and political . . . free reign'.[67] Southey also advocated the humanising influences of religion, morality, and custom, particularly as asserted through a national church, in bettering the conditions of the poor,[68] and he collaborated with Gooch in support of the 'Protestant Sisters of Charity' as a way to both improve care for the sick poor and to reaffirm the constitutional authority of the Church of England in the eyes of the lower classes.[69] This built upon his own longstanding interest in the Beguines, shared with his friend John Rickman.[70]

In a letter to Gooch in November 1814, Southey requested the Yarmouth Hospital anecdote for an article he was preparing for the *Quarterly* on the *Reports of the Society for Bettering the Conditions of the Poor*, explaining that his object is to 'show what has been done in this country towards lessening the quantum of human suffering, & what remains to do', and notes that 'schools, prisons, & hospitals' will all need to be addressed.[71] Southey did not use the anecdote in his review, which appeared in April 1816, although he does endorse 'societies like the Beguines of Flanders, and the *Sœurs de la Charité* of France' for their humanity and good works and includes another anecdote provided by Gooch to illustrate the connection between the 'absence of religion' and 'moral depravity', which he believed was at the heart of the 'condition of England' problem.[72] When the Yarmouth Hospital anecdote did appear in *Blackwood's*, Southey wrote to Gooch: 'It is not surprising that your letter in Blackwood should have produced so much impression. The subject comes home to everybody, & that Yarmouth story is one of the most touching incidents I ever remember to have heard.'[73] As Gooch relays to Blackwood in January 1826, the '"Sisters of Charity" was copied into several newspapers and recommended for adoption, and has produced a letter to the Bishop of London on the subject'.[74] Ultimately the project faltered,[75] but Southey's praise of Gooch's rhetorical affect is telling: the *Colloquies* were to be decried by Macaulay in the *Edinburgh Review* as an utterly unscientific production of 'taste and feeling'.[76]

As David M. Craig has shown, Southey was at the forefront of the conservative critique of political economy as the unfeeling science.[77] In a letter to Gooch in August 1829, he declares: 'As for the Political Economists, no words can express the thorough contempt which I feel for them. They discard all moral considerations from their philosophy, – & in their practice they have no compassion for flesh & blood.'[78] In this sentiment he was actually far more in tune with *Blackwood's* than with the liberal (Canningite) Toryism that predominated (albeit not to the exclusion of other forms of conservatism) in the *Quarterly* in the 1820s.[79] In the *Colloquies* the political economists are derided as immoral and irreligious,[80] while the medical profession is endorsed as a modern profession capable of supporting a paternalistic church and state – but only if medical education is 'a school of Christian humanity', for, according to Southey, 'when it is not so, the profession which of all others ought most to soften the heart, tends sureliest [sic] to corrupt and harden it'.[81] This 'bad doctor' narrative mirrors the alleged heartlessness of the political economists, in contrast to the recuperative potential of a moral economy endorsed by Christian medical practitioners.

Southey's friend Gooch, whom he considered 'one of the most remarkable men of his time',[82] appears to have been a leading candidate. In May 1829, he writes to Gooch regarding the pleasure he would feel if Gooch became a 'voluminous author', for 'not in any

way can you do so much good'.[83] As Southey explains to Rickman
in July 1829, 'Gooch is one of those persons who is zealous in the
right way.'[84] Beyond Southey's continued support for the Protestant
Sisters of Charity, Gooch, Southey, and Rickman together discussed
the social good that might be affected by co-operative societies, cultivation of waste lands, and colonisation, and Gooch published an
article on the co-operative society in Brighton in the *Quarterly* in
November 1829.[85] Their final letters address the proposed religious
order of nurses. After failing to interest the Bishop of London in
the project, Gooch and Southey, along with the Evangelical minister
Alexander Dallas, worked to gain the support of Elizabeth Fry and
Amelia Opie. However, it was the Reverend J. J. Hornby, Rector
of Warwick, who rallied to the cause, drawing upon Gooch's proposed scheme to supply the Liverpool infirmary with 'a better class
of nurses'.[86] In December 1829 Southey transcribes a letter he has
received from Hornby for Gooch. Hornby, working to gain the support of Southey, writes, '(I owe I have the pleasure of announcing;
and, I am pretty sure you will be gratified to hear) that the measure originates within the bosom of the established Church.' He also
wishes to be brought into communication with Gooch so that he
can ask his advice on 'the quantum of medical knowledge it will be
practical to give our nurses and the extent to which we may ~~cultivate~~
authorize them in exercising it'.[87] Gooch, perhaps due to worsening
health, was clearly hesitant, and in the final extant letter from the
poet, Southey pets his ego, noting that Hornby has 're-printed your
letter from Blackwood & the Med: Gazette for gratuitous distribu-
tion' and encouragingly declaring, 'This is a wicked world Gooch,
but there are good men enough in it to make a good fight, & ~~xx~~ win
it too, if they will exert themselves, everyone in his way, & stand by
each other.'[88] In the immediate aftermath of Gooch's death, Southey
writes of his friend, 'Never was man more desirous of doing all in his
power towards diminishing the sum of human misery,' and a perusal
of Southey's extant correspondence indicates that it was Gooch's
keen moral sense, Christian humanity, and zeal, along with his literary talents and good taste, that made him such a valued friend.[89]

   As Michelle Faubert has observed, Coleridge includes the 'sages'
of 'medicine and physiology' as part of the 'CLERISY of the nation,
or national church'.[90] This inclusion is underlined by Coleridge's use
of a medical metaphor in the advertisement to his work, in which

he compares its dictates to a physician's 'medicine and the method of cure'.[91] A master metaphor of contagion pervades Southey's *Colloquies* as well as his contributions to the *Quarterly*: political radicalism, unrest and irreligion are collectively depicted as contagious diseases spread by the popular press, while the 'greedy spirit of trade' is 'an epidemic malady in this land'.[92] The metaphor was derived from the ongoing debate on the contagious nature of diseases, figured in the popular periodical press as a battle between conservative contagionists and Benthamite anti-contagionists, who saw quarantine as an impediment to commercial progress and a product of despotic governments, to which Gooch was a key contributor.[93] With the 'condition of England' problem cast in the figurative language of disease, it was only logical that medical figures would be envisioned as part of the cure.

The publication of Henry Southey's sketch in *Lives of British Physicians* in late July 1830 solidified Gooch's public persona following his early death on 16th February 1830.[94] In the public sensation that accompanied the publication of Warren's *Passages from the Diary of a Late Physician* in August 1830, some readers suspected that 'the late Dr. Gooch's papers had afforded the materials' for the series.[95] His known connection to the magazine and the coincidental timing of his death surely fed the rumour. The inclusion of extracts from Gooch's 'loose papers' and manuscript letters, written in the first person, may also have contributed, and the Gothic imagery of some passages is not unlike that used by the late physician. Recalling his study of 'a whole articulated skeleton' in his room when a young apprentice, he writes that, one night, 'I shut my eyes, and began to forget myself, when, whether I was aware or asleep, or between both, I cannot tell – but suddenly I felt two bony hands grasp my ancles [sic], and pull me down the bed; if it had been real it could not have been more distinct. For some time, how long, I cannot tell, I almost fainted with terror.'[96] The Gothic provides a language of intensely embodied affect that indicates a sustained receptiveness to the 'feeling of common humanity' in the face of the horrors faced by the medical professional.[97]

More broadly, Gooch and others constructed his public persona within the same ideological matrix as the late physician. Within this matrix, the traditional moral economy of eighteenth-century Scottish medicine – 'the pre-modern, medieval, Scottish Highland, moral-aristocratic concept of paternalism' associated with Gregory's medical ethics and 'the fiduciary concept of medicine as a profession that it helped to create'[98] – was discursively deployed against Scotch political economy and, in tandem, against the perceived irreligion and heartlessness of the medical profession in the early nineteenth century. This deployment served the agenda of Romantic conservatism while also contributing to a public relations campaign for the medical profession. Gooch's friend Robert Ferguson, founding editor of the *London Medical Gazette*, prolific man of letters, and physician-extraordinary to Queen Victoria, was a leading figure in both movements, and first made his entrance onto the literary stage via *Blackwood's*.

Robert Ferguson: The Medical Clerisy and a Counter-Example in the *Quarterly*

In a contribution to the 'Horæ Germanicæ' series for *Blackwood's* in September 1824, which marks the beginning of his long career as a contributor to the popular periodical press, Ferguson opens by praising the Catholic scholarship of the Germans: '[r]egarding philosophy, poetry, the arts and sciences, as productions of mind, they have never imagined that the knowledge of one of these necessarily excluded that of any of the others'.[99] While admitting the truth of 'the homely adage, that to be "Jack of many trades, is to be master of none"', Ferguson explains:

> When the world require a close and studious devotion to any pursuit or profession, we feel that their claims are perfectly reasonable; but they are unreasonable only when they suppose that the EXERCISE in one branch of knowledge is totally incompatible with a thorough acquaintance with the PRINCIPLES of every other.[100]

This statement captures Ferguson's own lifelong practice as what today would be referred to as an 'interdisciplinary' thinker. For example, three decades later, in a review of Brodie's *Psychological Inquiries* (1854) for the *Quarterly Review*, Ferguson affirms that 'in future no one has any right to discuss a metaphysical question as to the nature of the intellectual powers who neglects to master the results of modern physiology'.[101] The close link between philosophy and medicine for Ferguson reflects his Edinburgh training.[102] By the mid-nineteenth century, however, not everyone looked favourably upon his elite literary eclecticism. An obituary in *The Lancet* notes that the 'courtly' Ferguson 'looked upon his own profession as one that was hardly good enough for him',[103] while an obituary in the *Medical Times and Gazette* defends him against the charge of being an 'idle, haphazard, mere fashionable Doctor which, as he said, some of his contemporaries were pleased to call him'.[104] Ferguson regarded his zeal for 'whatever there was most intellectual in the world of letters' as well as in 'physic'[105] as a vital component of his role as one of the medical clerisy:

> that man, who, having disciplined his mind with 'all the knowledge of the Egyptians,' and having extracted from it the principles upon which that knowledge is grounded, gives his nights and days to any one pursuit, is far more likely to become a benefactor to the human race, than he who has studied only one thing.[106]

While the discussion of Lessing's *Laocoon, or, the limits of Poetry and Painting* (1766) which follows brings Ferguson's medical reasoning to bear upon a question of ancient Greek aesthetics, his broader corpus of popular periodical writings draws upon his extensive medical, literary, historical, and philosophical reading to explore a range of pertinent medical and social questions, including lighter fare, such as the lessons the physician might learn from studying Shakespeare (in a highly complimentary review of that most aristocratic of physicians, Sir Henry Halford), as well as more pressing issues, such as the influence of civilization on public health, the contagious nature of cholera and appropriate governmental responses, the connection between public health and mortality rates, and the best ways to reform the regulation of mines and prisons.[107]

Ferguson's contributions to the debates on public health offer a key contrast to those of Alison and Gooch. Like Alison's, his writings express concerns regarding the health of the urban poor, and while writing of the 'miseries of Glasgow' in a review on 'Public Health and Mortality' for the *Quarterly* in June 1840, he notes his 'regret that the work of Dr. Alison, on the Poor of Scotland, had not reached us in time to use his facts on the present occasion', as '[i]t is one of the most interesting volumes that we ever perused, worthy of a consummate physician, and kind and tender-hearted friend of the poor'.[108] Ferguson also endorses Alison's campaign for a Scottish poor law in a review of 'Colliers and Collieries' in June 1842, written in support of Lord Ashley's proposal for a bill to regulate the age and sex of children and young persons employed in mines and collieries.[109] What is lacking is the rhetorical affect cultivated by Alison and Gooch. In his article on 'Colliers and Collieries', Ferguson appeals to the miserable conditions of the mines and their effect on children's minds and bodies, and refers to the '*terrible* woodcuts' that accompany the *Report of the Commissioners for Inquiring into the Condition of Children employed in Mines, &c. with two Appendices of Evidence* (1842).[110] However, the grand conclusion of the piece, which announces that since first drafting this review Lord Ashley's bill has received the unanimous support of the House of Commons, is not that natural humanity has prevailed, but rather that 'the danger of neglecting the moral and social and also the physical condition of the poor in this rich and powerful empire has at length been understood and appreciated'.[111] Underplaying the sentimental force of Ashley's speech, Ferguson concludes that members of the House, rather than being moved by his oratory,

> felt, we hope and believe, that this was the first step in a path which must be pursued, if our working classes – unequalled in history of the world for courage, energy, and native goodness of feeling – are to be reconciled to the great existing institutions of their country.[112]

Similarly, in 'Public Health and Mortality', Ferguson supports the argument for sanitary reform by appealing to the risks posed to the wealthy, both from the spread of infection ('if man will not be linked to man by sympathy of feeling, most assuredly he shall be by the bonds of suffering and disease') and from the increase in poor rates that would result from epidemic disease.[113] If Alison and Gooch built upon the 'neo-Mackenzian revival of "feeling"' associated with *Blackwood's* in developing and popularising their political medicine,[114] Ferguson's writings were more in keeping with the ideology of the *Quarterly*.

In Frank W. Fetter's summary, '[t]he idea that the landed gentry were the bulwark of stable government, the support of the established church, and the foundation of education, was the premise of much of the economic argument in the two Tory journals'; however, *Blackwood's* was distinctive in that '[t]here was a humour, and at the same time a humanitarianism, that made its language, and sometimes its policies, differ from that of the *Quarterly*'.[115] Generalisations about either periodical can of course be problematic. For example, G. Poulett Scrope, a major contributor to the *Quarterly* on poor laws between 1835 and 1844, wrote in support of outdoor relief in Ireland in 1845 but was then contradicted in a subsequent article by Mortimore O'Sullivan: 'We give Mr. Poulett Scrope credit for most sincere humanity; but he is a man of lively imagination, and the extent to which he has become blind to the plainest facts in this case is truly lamentable.'[116] Even the humanity of Scrope, however, had to be subservient to the need to maintain social order. Writing against Chalmers' idealisation of virtuous poverty, he declares:

> the question to this extent was long ago determined in the minds of all whose humanity is directed by judgment, and who, instead of dwelling with pleasure on the sentimental picture of one starving being sharing his last crust or potato with another, desire, not merely in the interests of humanity, but likewise for the sake of the peace, order, and morality of society, that the property of the country should be made responsible for preventing the existence of extreme destitution, or its only alternative, permitted mendicancy and vagrancy.[117]

If the primary rhetoric in *Blackwood's* is that of natural humanity and Christian duty, the writers in the *Quarterly* continually return to the need to quell the discontent of the working classes – to alleviate conditions that 'unloose every social tie, and excite the outburst of the most savage, desperate, and demoniac passions' – in the name of social stability.[118]

An apt comparison is between Wilson on 'The Factory System' in *Blackwood's* and Lord Ashley on 'The Factory System' (1836) and 'Infant Labour' (1840) in the *Quarterly*. Ashley does make exclamations 'in the name of humanity and of God', but opens his article on 'The Factory System' with an acknowledgement of the threat the system presents not only to the 'honour', but also 'perhaps the safety, of the empire' and the potential 'danger, in revealing to a mighty mass the multitude of their fellow sufferers, and the extent of their

wrongs'.[119] Wilson, in contrast, opens with an evocation of the importance of charity, which 'is but another name for love', and a diatribe
against the factory system's disregard for the bodies and souls of
workers. Throughout his essay Wilson insists that 'life is more than
the meat' and the industrial classes 'have minds – and what is more,
hearts, and immortal souls'.[120] If he has any fears, it is for the degradation of 'national character' in the lower orders, namely the Scotch
peasantry, which, according to his earlier essay, 'Some Observations
on the Poetry of the Agricultural and that of the Pastoral Districts in
Scotland' (1819), spawned the likes of Burns and Hogg – the peasantry who, 'simple and pure in their morals – tender and affectionate
in their hearts', enabled 'a spirit of poetry' to breathe across all the
valleys of Scotland.[121] The factory system 'by its unnatural labours,
dulls and deadens those affections in the hearts of the poor' which
are the foundations of the traditional paternalistic society so valued
by *Blackwood's*.[122] Ashley similarly writes that the worker needs
'time and opportunity for the cultivation and exercise of his immortal part', but only after expressing his concern that currently 'the
minds of the people are left in total darkness, to be illuminated at
intervals only by the livid and unwholesome glare of infidelity and
sedition'.[123] Again, in 'Infant Labour', Ashley justifies the need to
regulate child labour by appealing to fears of revolutionary uprising –
the 'two great demons' of 'Socialism and Chartism' – and 'the vast
and inflammable mass which lies waiting, day by day, for the spark
to explode it into mischief'.[124] To provide another point of comparison: when W. R. Greg writes on 'Juvenile and Female Labour'
in the *Edinburgh Review* in January 1844, he aims his attempt 'to
awaken some sympathy' for the industrious classes towards what he
sees as the underlying problems – 'the *ignorance* and *redundancy* of
our population; or, to speak more correctly; the neglect of popular
instruction, and the limitation of the field of employment by corrupt
and selfish laws'.[125] The remedies are not the interventionist legislative changes promoted by Wilson and Ashley but rather free trade –
'unshackled industry and unrestricted commerce' – and popular
education that not only teaches 'the cultivation of religious feelings,
the explanation of religious truth, and the inculcation of moral and
social duties' but also, unsurprisingly, political economy.[126]

Surrounded by these transauthorial discourses, it is perhaps
unsurprising that Ferguson's contributions to the debates on the

poor law and sanitary and factory reform in the *Quarterly* do not promote the same recuperative medical humanism as Gooch and Alison in the Blackwoodian context. Had Ferguson contributed to *Blackwood's* on these issues, it is likely he would have framed his argument differently. Gooch, for example, in 'Protestant Sisters of Charity', writes in a mode utterly distinct from his contributions to the *Quarterly*. His description of his friend the 'country clergy-man', who with a 'warm and tender heart' finds happiness in dutiful service, echoes the character of George Robert Gleig's 'The Coun-try Curate', first introduced in *Blackwood's* one month prior to the publication of Gooch's manifesto, while his own self-characterisa-tion as a medical man of feeling, 'affected' with a 'pang of self-reproach' by the unnecessary death of a patient who had 'excited unusual interest', looks forward the voice of the late physician.[127] In contrast to this emotive (and more inherently 'literary') rhetoric, Gooch's article on 'Contagion and Quarantine' for the *Quarterly* in July 1822 is intended to provide 'a fair opportunity for the exer-cise of unfettered comparison and unbiassed [sic] judgment', and he prefaces his rebuttal to the anti-contagionists in the *Quarterly* in December 1825 with a declaration that he will not extract 'distress-ing' scenes of the London plague of 1665, recorded by Dr Nathaniel Hodges, lest he be 'accused of desiring to interest the feelings of our readers in the opening of a most important inquiry, when it is and ought to be our intention only to appeal to their judgments'.[128] Such a declaration would be utterly out of place in *Blackwood's*, though Gooch does resort to *Blackwood's* to publish a continuation of his article on the plague, in a similarly staid voice, after '[t]he Editor's pruning hook was so freely used on my article on the plague in the Quarterly that I have committed an act of injustice to the author whom I profess to review'.[129]

Ferguson's early contributions to *Blackwood's* are in a different mode entirely from his articles in the *Quarterly*, generally focusing more on literary than on medical topics (though, in the case of his discussion of Lessing's *Laocoon*, drawing upon medical 'principles') and also ranging into short fiction. His two-part 'Letters from the Continent', although based on his sojourn in Germany as a student just prior to beginning medical school at Edinburgh, largely eschew medical subject-matter, with the exception of a critique of profes-sional society in England, where 'John Bull thinks it incumbent upon himself always to carry the outward and visible signs of his pursuits at the mast-head', such that if

> you see a face, which nature intended to be merry, trying to lodge as much wisdom on the thin pencil of its supercilia as would weigh down the penthouse of a Samuel Johnson, you guess that you are in contact with a young votary of Æsculapius.[130]

If Ferguson builds upon any Blackwoodian discourses, it is upon Moir's critique of professional culture. He founded the *London Medical Gazette* with the explicit purpose of promoting the 'philosophic views' and 'gentlemanlike feelings' in medical culture which the reforming polemics of *The Lancet* were seen to undermine.[131]

The Medical Blackwoodians: Preliminary Conclusions

Blackwood's provided a unique opportunity for Ferguson to experiment with a range of forms within an ideological context that in many ways stood opposed to emergent medico-scientific values in the nineteenth century. Like Delta, Ferguson insisted upon strict secrecy as to his authorship, and wrote to Blackwood in October 1824: '<u>Above all</u> I request that nobody not even Lockhart (whom I shall inform myself) may know my articles – It is of some consequence or I should not insist upon it.'[132] However, he also notes in a subsequent letter that 'In society I have heard many a young aspirant for literary honors Barists Doctor & laymen wishing to atchieve [sic] one article in <u>the</u> Blackwood.'[133] Such aspirations are in part due to the sheer cultural clout of Maga. However, the insistence on anonymity most likely reflects both the public's apparent suspicion of literary medical men and the magazine's polemical character. Gooch, for example, notes in a letter to Blackwood in 1826 that he likes and dislikes Maga in turn, finding the voice of the January 1826 preface and the *Noctes* 'a noisy, boisterous, coarse, vulgar wit', and warns that '[i]t has been, and still is the Prince of Magazines, and ought to be conducted with so much the more care because of the extensive influence it has on the public mind'.[134]

The benefits of this 'extensive influence' were reaped by both Gooch and Alison in promoting their humanistic political medicine, but they also benefited from and contributed to the particular ideological and discursive framing of the magazine. The reactionary Romantic ideology of *Blackwood's* emphasised a problematic disjunction between intellect and feeling – manifest in the outcry against not only the supposed materialism and scepticism of the *Edinburgh Review*, but also political economy, utilitarianism, and the 'march of intellect' more broadly. This included a 'bad doctor' narrative against which Gooch and Alison, along with Delta and Warren's late physician, acted as conservative correctives: members of a medical clerisy. If the 'medico-popular' tale of terror evolved from the case histories included in the early numbers (amongst other popular forms), moving subversively from the voice of an objective, authoritative author to a first-person narrator who has suffered psychological or physical trauma, medical contributors (and those who wished to be read as such) quickly reclaimed the genre, an act which culminated in Warren's late physician and spiralled into a new genre of medico-popular writing. While this reclamation was at times uneasy (as particularly illustrated by Macnish's writing), a magazine that could be and often was openly hostile to professional medical culture (particularly within its own city, Edinburgh) became instrumental in promoting a recuperative medical humanism that not only informed the construction of an idealised literary medical man for the wider nineteenth-century reading public and the creation of an enduring genre of popular medical writing, but also played a key role in the popular debates on the rise of public health policy in the first half of the nineteenth century.

Notes

1. [John Eagles], 'New Scheme for Maintaining the Poor. Poor-Law Sonnets', *BEM*, 43 (April 1838), 483–93 (p. 493).
2. Hamilton, *The Healers*, p. 197.
3. Hamlin, *Public Health and Social Justice*, pp. 215–16.
4. For a summation of this opposition, see Fetter, 'Economy Controversy in the British Reviews'. For a comparison of the *Edinburgh* versus the *Quarterly*, see Fetter, 'The Economic Articles in the *Quarterly Review* and Their Authors'. On *Blackwood's* and poor law economics, see Fetter, 'The Economic Articles in *Blackwood's Edinburgh Magazine* and their Authors'; Milne, *The Politics of Blackwood's*. For an examination of the political economy in the *Edinburgh*, see Fontana, *Rethinking the Politics of Commercial Society*.
5. Hamlin, *Public Health and Social Justice*, p. 3.

6. Milne, *The Politics of Blackwood's*, p. 424; Roberts, 'The Social Conscience of Tory Periodicals', p. 167.
7. Ibid.
8. [John Wilson], 'The Factory System', *BEM*, 33 (April 1833), 419–50 (p. 439).
9. Ibid. pp. 430–4. For a general discussion of the involvement of medical men in factory reform, see Gray, *The Factory Question and Industrial England*, pp. 72–85.
10. [Wilson], 'The Factory System', p. 420.
11. [John Wilson], 'On Poor's Laws, and their Introduction into Ireland', *BEM*, 33 (May 1833), 811–43 (p. 812).
12. [J. G. Lockhart], 'Political Economy', *BEM*, 12 (November 1822), 525–30; [Eagles], 'New Scheme for Maintaining the Poor'; [Henry Thomson], 'Panaceas for Poverty', *BEM*, 14 (December 1823), 635–8.
13. [John Eagles], 'Medical Attendance and Other Parochials. By A Curate, in a Letter to a Friend', *BEM*, 41 (May 1837), 629–42 (p. 632).
14. Martin, *William Pulteney Alison*, p. 199. Alison's relationship to the Blackwood publishing house spans the length of his career and may have been guided by the close relationship that his younger brother, Archibald Alison (1792–1867), maintained with the Blackwoods. On Archibald Alison, see Milne, 'Archibald Alison: Conservative Controversialist'; Michie, *An Enlightenment Tory in Victorian Scotland*, pp. 159–97.
15. Alison's argument is summarised in [Charles Neaves], 'Highland Destitution', *BEM*, 62 (November 1847), 630–42.
16. Alison, *Observations on the Management of the Poor in Scotland*, p. v.
17. Ibid. p. 73. On Alison's public debate with Chalmers, see Checkland, 'Chalmers and William Pulteney Alison'.
18. Alison, *Observations on the Management of the Poor in Scotland*, p. 104.
19. For further, see Hamlin, 'William Pulteney Alison, the Scottish Philosophy, and the Making of a Political Medicine'.
20. [W. P. Alison], 'Evils of the State of Ireland,' *BEM*, 40 (October 1836), 495–514 (p. 495, p. 499, p. 500).
21. [Wilson], 'On Poor's Laws, and their Introduction into Ireland', p. 822.
22. For example, see: [Thomas Spring-Rice], 'Proposed Introduction of Poor Laws into Ireland', ER, 59 (April 1834), 227–61; 'Monypenny on the Scottish Poor Laws', *ER*, 59 (July 1834), 425–38; [Edwin

Chadwick], 'The New Poor Laws', *ER*, 63 (July 1836), 487–537; [W. B. Wrightson], 'The Workhouse System – The Irish Poor Bill', *ER*, 66 (October 1837), 186–208.

23. [Henry Reeve], 'Inquiry into the State of the Poor', *ER*, 11 (October 1807), 100–15 (p. 104).
24. [Alison], 'Evils of the State of Ireland', p. 495, p. 501.
25. [Wilson], 'The Factory System', p. 420, p. 423.
26. Ibid. p. 444.
27. [Lockhart], *Peter's Letters to his Kinsfolk*, vol. 1, p. 176.
28. [Alison], 'Justice to Ireland', p. 817.
29. [Alison], 'On the Miseries of Ireland, and their Remedies', p. 658; Hamlin, 'William Pulteney Alison, the Scottish Philosophy, and the Making of a Political Medicine', p. 162, p. 184.
30. [Alison], 'On the Miseries of Ireland, and their Remedies', p. 658.
31. *The Liverpool Mercury* (1 July 1831), Issue 1052.
32. 'To What Miseries are not the Poor Exposed?', *Kaleidoscope; or, Literary and Scientific Mirror*, 11 (5 July 1831), 420–2 (p. 421).
33. Ibid. p. 421.
34. [Samuel Warren], 'Passages from the Diary of a Late Physician. Chap. X. A Slight Cold – Rich and Poor – Grave Doings', *BEM*, 29 (June 1831), 946–67 (p. 960, p. 959).
35. Hamlin, *Public Health and Social Justice*, p. 165, p. 170.
36. Ibid. p. 201, p. 208.
37. As Hamlin notes in regard to the medical men (with the exception of Alison) who contributed to the *Local Reports*, 'A good deal of the subhumanness reporters attributed to their subjects resulted directly from their inability to imagine how people existed in such situations' (ibid. p. 212).
38. For an overview, see Ledger, 'Radical Writing', pp. 127–46.
39. [Alison], 'Evils of the State of Ireland', p. 513.
40. See Hilary Marland, 'Gooch, Robert (1784–1830)', in *ODNB*, available at http://www.oxforddnb.com/view/article/10940 (last accessed 20 June 2016); 'Robert Gooch, M.D.', in Munk, *The Roll of the Royal College of Physicians of London*, pp. 100–5.
41. Cutmore, *Contributors to the Quarterly Review*, p. 94. This view was not, however, unchallenged. See A. B. Granville, 'The Late Doctor Gooch and his Biographers', *LMG*, 7 (23 October 1830), 104–7. Gooch also wrote directly to Sir Robert Peel regarding the proposed reform of quarantine laws and received an interested response. See, Robert Gooch to Robert Peel, 17 April 1825, © The British Library Board, Add. 40376, fols 301–2 and Robert Peel to Robert Gooch, 26 June 1825, © The British Library Board, Add. 40379, fol. 207.

42. Richardson, *Death, Dissection and the Destitute*, p. 166, p. 176, p. 185.
43. Robert Gooch to John Murray, 30 September 1829, NLS MS 40458.
44. [Henry Herbert Southey], 'Gooch', in *Lives of British Physicians*, p. 338.
45. Robert Gooch to John Murray, no date [1830], NLS MS 40458.
46. Marland, 'Gooch, Robert (1784–1830)' in *ODNB*.
47. Ibid.; 'Robert Gooch, M.D.', in Munk, *The Roll of the Royal College of Physicians of London*, pp. 101–3, and [Southey], 'Gooch', in *Lives of British Physicians*, pp. 305–41.
48. [Southey], 'Gooch', in *Lives of British Physicians*, p. 319.
49. Robert Southey to John Murray, 15 February 1812, in Ian Packer and Lynda Pratt (eds), *The Collected Letters of Robert Southey, Part Four: 1810–1815, Romantic Circles Electronic Edition*, available at http://www.rc.umd.edu/editions/southey_letters/Part_Four/HTML/letterEEd.26.2039.html (last accessed 20 June 2016).
50. Robert Southey to John Murray, 31 January 1813, in ibid., available at http://www.rc.umd.edu/editions/southey_letters/Part_Four/HTML/letterEEd.26.2214.html (last accessed 20 June 2016).
51. Southey did facilitate a contribution to the *Edinburgh Annual Register, for 1810*. See Robert Southey to Robert Gooch, 10 June 1811, in ibid., available at http://www.rc.umd.edu/editions/southey_letters/Part_Four/HTML/letterEEd.26.1934.html (last accessed 20 June 2016). This contribution was [Robert Gooch], 'Life of Dr Beddoes', *Edinburgh Annual Register, for 1810*, Vol Third – Part Second (Edinburgh: Printed for John Ballantyne and Co., for John Ballantyne and Co. Edinburgh; Longman, Hurst, Rees, Orme, and Brown; and John Murray, London, 1812), pp. 516–37. The appearance of his first article in the *Quarterly* may also have been facilitated by John Taylor Coleridge, whose wife Gooch attended. In a letter to Coleridge, Gooch thanks him for his 'offer to present my article' and notes that it is not 'too scientific' and 'popular enough and long enough for the Editor's pruning'. (Robert Gooch to John Taylor Coleridge, 19 December 1821, © The British Library Board, Add. 86233).
52. Robert Ferguson to William Blackwood, [1825?], NLS MS 4014, fols 216–17.
53. Robert Gooch to William Blackwood, 28 November 1825, NLS MS 4014, fols 272–3.
54. Robert Southey to Robert Gooch, 15 December 1811, in *The Collected Letters of Robert Southey, Part Four*, available at http://www.rc.umd.edu/editions/southey_letters/Part_Four/HTML/letterEEd.26.1999.html (last accessed 20 June 2016).

55. [Robert Gooch], 'Two Days with Dr. Parr', *BEM*, 18 (November 1825), 596–601 (p. 599).

56. [Robert Gooch], 'Protestant Sisters of Charity', *BEM*, 18 (December 1825), 732–5 (p. 732).

57. Ibid. pp. 732–3.

58. Haakonssen, *Medicine and Morals in the Enlightenment*, p. 27. See also Wild, 'The Origins of a Modern Medical Ethics in Enlightenment Scotland', in Coyer and Shuttleton (eds), *Scottish Medicine and Literary Culture*, pp. 48–73.

59. [Gooch], 'Protestant Sisters of Charity', p. 734.

60. Ibid. p. 734.

61. D. M. Moir to William Blackwood, 20 November [1825?], NLS MS 4015, fols 98–9.

62. [Gooch], 'Protestant Sisters of Charity', p. 734.

63. Christie, '*Blackwood's Edinburgh Magazine* in the Scientific Culture of Early Nineteenth-Century Edinburgh', in Morrison and Roberts (eds), *Romanticism and Blackwood's Magazine*, pp. 125–36.

64. [Robert Gooch], 'Medical Attendance on the Country Poor' *LMG*, 1 (12 January 1828), 151–4 (p. 153).

65. [Robert Gooch], 'Medical Attendance on the Country Poor', *LMG*, 1 (22 December 1827), 55–8 (p. 56).

66. Eastwood, 'Robert Southey and the Intellectual Origins of Romantic Conservativism', p. 327.

67. Southey, *Colloquies*, vol. 1, p. 56.

68. In addition to the *Colloquies*, see [Robert Southey], 'Inquiry into the Poor Laws, &c.', *QR*, 8 (December 1812), 319–56 and [Robert Southey], 'The Poor', *QR*, 15 (April 1816), 187–235.

69. On this missionary aspect of the project, see [Dallas], *Protestant Sisters of Charity*, pp. 9–10.

70. His interest in the Beguines dates at least to 1800. See Robert Southey to John Rickman, 9 January 1800, in Ian Packer and Lynda Pratt (eds), *The Collected Letters of Robert Southey, Part Two: 1798–1803, Romantic Circles Electronic Edition*, available at http://www.rc.umd. edu/editions/southey_letters/Part_Two/HTML/letterEEd.26.476.html (last accessed 20 June 2016). Southey supported Gooch by sharing his previous research on the Beguines. See Robert Southey to Robert Gooch, 18 December 1825, Bodleian Libraries, University of Oxford, Don d. 86, fols 15–16.

71. Robert Southey to Robert Gooch, 30 November 1814, in *The Collected Letters of Robert Southey, Part Four*, available at http://www.rc.umd. edu/editions/southey_letters/Part_Four/HTML/letterEEd.26.2507. html (last accessed 20 June 2016).

72. [Southey], 'The Poor', p. 229, pp. 232–3. On the source of the anecdote, see Robert Southey to Sharon Turner, 2 April 1816, in Charles Cuthbert Southey (ed.), *The Life and Correspondence of Robert Southey*, vol. 4, p. 157.

73. Robert Southey to Robert Gooch, 18 December 1825, Bodleian Libraries, University of Oxford, Don d. 86, fol. 15.

74. Robert Gooch to William Blackwood, 2 January 1826, NLS MS 4017, fols 101–2.

75. For a detailed overview, see Perry Williams, 'Religion, respectability and the origins of the modern nurse', in French and Wear (eds), *British Medicine in an Age of Reform*, pp. 231–55.

76. [Thomas Macaulay], 'Southey's Colloquies on Society', *ER*, 50 (January 1830), 528–65 (p. 533).

77. Craig, *Robert Southey and Romantic Apostasy*, pp. 166–88.

78. Robert Southey to Robert Gooch, 8 August 1829, Bodleian Libraries, University of Oxford, Don d. 86, fol. 31.

79. For an overview of the politics of the *Quarterly*, see Cutmore, 'Introduction', in Cutmore (ed.), *Conservativism and the Quarterly Review*, pp. 1–18. On Southey's deviations from the official line taken by the *Quarterly*, see Hilton, '"Sardonic Grins" and "Paranoid Politics"' and Speck, 'Robert Southey's Contribution to the *Quarterly Review*', in Cutmore (ed.), *Conservativism and the Quarterly Review*, pp. 41–60 (p. 53), pp. 165–77.

80. See for example Southey, *Colloquies*, vol. 2, p. 261.

81. Ibid. p. 319.

82. 'Robert Gooch, M.D.', in Munk, *The Roll of the Royal College of Physicians of London*, p. 103.

83. Robert Southey to Robert Gooch, 19 May 1829, Bodleian Libraries, University of Oxford, Don d. 86, fol. 26.

84. Robert Southey to John Rickman, 16 July 1829, in Warter (ed.), *Selections from the Letters of Robert Southey*, vol. 4, p. 142.

85. See Story, *Robert Southey: A Life*, pp. 318–19; [Robert Gooch], 'The Co-operatives', *QR*, 41 (November 1829), 359–75.

86. Robert Southey to Robert Gooch, 3 December 1829, Bodleian Libraries, University of Oxford, Don d. 86, fols 33–4.

87. Ibid.

88. Robert Southey to Robert Gooch, 18 January 1830, Bodleian Libraries, University of Oxford, Don d. 86, fols 36–7.

89. Robert Southey to Mrs Hodson, 16 March 1830, in Charles Cuthbert Southey (ed.), *The Life and Correspondence of Robert Southey*, vol. 6, p. 93. Throughout his letters to various correspondents, Southey references Gooch's literary tastes, and for example, when composing

his epic poem, *Roderick, the Last of the Goths* (1814), he wrote to his brother Henry that 'Gooch is one of the few persons whom *I wish to see it.*' (Robert Southey to Henry Herbert Southey, 4 November 1812, in *The Collected Letters of Robert Southey, Part Four,* available at http://www.rc.umd.edu/editions/southey_letters/Part_Four/HTML/letterEEd.26.2173.html (last accessed 20 June 2016).)

90. Coleridge, *On the Constitution of Church and State*, vol. 10, p. 46, as cited by Faubert, *Rhyming Reason*, p. 25. As Faubert notes, Roy Porter has likewise written that '[Thomas] Beddoes's vision of the doctor as intellectual guru parallels Coleridge's ideal of the new intelligentsia, the clerisy, called to serve as moral leaders of the future' (*Doctor of Society: Thomas Beddoes and the Sick Trade in Late-Enlightenment England* (London: Routledge, 1992), p. 190, as cited by Faubert, *Rhyming Reason*, p. 205 (note 93)).

91. Coleridge, *On the Constitution of Church and State*, p. iv.

92. Southey, *Colloquies*, vol. 2, p. 255. A few examples of this metaphor regarding radicalism, scepticism, and unrest and the popular press may be found in vol. 2, p. 42, p. 110, and p. 172. On Southey's medical metaphors, see Budge, 'Medicine, the "manufacturing system," and Southey's Romantic conservativism'.

93. For a detailed reading, see Connell, *Romanticism, Economics, and the Question of 'Culture'*, pp. 247–57.

94. An advertisement announcing publication 'on Monday next' may be found in *The Literary Gazette: A weekly journal of literature, science, and the fine arts*, 704 (17 July 1830), 472. The text is in the 'List of New Works' section in the *MM*, 10 (August 1830), 238 and is reviewed in *The Monthly Review*, 14 (August 1830), 600–12.

95. William Blackwood to Samuel Warren, postmarked 23 February 1831, NLS MS 4732, fols 15–16.

96. [Southey], 'Gooch', in *Lives of British Physicians*, p. 306, p. 307. Other examples of Gothic imagery include a letter on the 'unearthly scene' of the Beguines in chapel at Ghent (p. 336) and his own terror of lecturing (p. 324).

97. Moir, *The Modern Pythagorean*, vol. 1, p. 123.

98. McCullough, *John Gregory and the Invention of Professional Medical Ethics*, pp. 291–2.

99. [Robert Ferguson], 'Horæ Germanicæ. No. XVIII. Lessing's Laocoon, or, the Limits of Poetry and Painting', *BEM*, 16 (September 1824), 312–16 (p. 312).

100. Ibid. p. 312.

101. [Robert Ferguson], 'Psychological inquiries', *QR*, 96 (December 1854), 86–117 (p. 105).

102. For an overview of links between medicine and philosophy in Scotland, see Hamlin, 'William Pulteney Alison, the Scottish Philosophy, and the Making of a Political Medicine', pp. 168–9.

103. 'Dr. Robert Ferguson', *The Lancet* (1 July 1865), 25.

104. 'Robert Ferguson', *Medical Times and Gazette* (1 July 1865), 13–15 (p. 15).

105. Ibid. p. 13.

106. [Ferguson], 'Horæ Germanicæ', p. 312.

107. [Robert Ferguson], 'Sir Henry Halford's *Essays*', QR, 49 (April 1833), 175–98; [Robert Ferguson], 'Berard – *Influence of Civilization on Public Health*', *Foreign Quarterly Review*, 1 (July 1827), 178–88; [Robert Ferguson], 'The Cholera', QR, 46 (November 1831), 169–212; [Robert Ferguson], 'Directions of the Privy Council in Case of Pestilence', QR, 46 (November 1831), 264–73; [Robert Ferguson], 'Public Health and Mortality', QR, 66 (June 1840), 115–55; [Robert Ferguson], 'Colliers and Collieries', QR, 70 (June 1842), 158–95; [Robert Ferguson], 'Pentonville Prisoners', QR, 82 (December 1847), 175–206; [Robert Ferguson], 'The Two Systems at Pentonville', QR, 92 (March 1853), 487–506.

108. [Ferguson], 'Public Health and Mortality', p. 121.

109. [Ferguson], 'Colliers and Collieries', p. 191.

110. Ibid. p. 194.

111. Ibid. p. 194.

112. Ibid. p. 194.

113. [Ferguson], 'Public Health and Mortality', p. 123.

114. Duncan, *Scott's Shadow*, p. 226.

115. Fetter, 'Economy Controversy in the British Reviews', p. 431, p. 427.

116. [Mortimore O'Sullivan], 'Out-door Relief', QR, 79 (March 1847), 463–84 (p. 478). For further on Scrope in the *Quarterly*, see Fetter, 'The Economic Articles in the *Quarterly Review* and Their Authors', pp. 56–9.

117. [G. Poulett Scrope], 'Poor Laws for Scotland', QR, 75 (December 1844), 125–48 (p. 135).

118. [G. Poulett Scrope], 'Foreign Poor-Laws – Irish Poverty', QR, 55 (December 1835), 35–73 (p. 55). To be clear, *Blackwood's* was also concerned with the threat of a discontented labouring class. See for example [Charles Neaves], 'Discontents of the Working Classes', *BEM*, 43 (April 1838), 421–36, and [Robert Sowler], 'Revolt of the Workers. The Employer and the Employed', *BEM*, 52 (November 1842), 642–53. What I am referring to is a general rhetorical emphasis within public health articles.

119. [Anthony Ashley Cooper], 'The Factory System', QR, 57 (December 1836), 396–443 (p. 398, p. 396, p. 397).

120. [Wilson], 'The Factory System', p. 419, p. 434, p. 446.

121. [Wilson], 'On Poor's Laws', p. 814; [John Wilson], 'Some Observations on the Poetry of the Agricultural and that of the Pastoral Districts in Scotland, Illustrated by a Comparative View of the Genius of Burns and the Ettrick Shepherd', *BEM*, 4 (February 1819), 521–9 (p. 522).

122. [Wilson], 'The Factory System', p. 433.

123. [Anthony Ashley Cooper], 'The Factory System', p. 442.

124. [Anthony Ashley Cooper], 'Infant Labour', *QR*, 67 (December 1840), 171–81 (p. 180).

125. [W. R. Greg], 'Juvenile and Female Labour', *ER*, 79 (January 1844), 130–56 (p. 148, p. 151).

126. Ibid. p. 152, p. 155.

127. [Gooch], 'Protestant Sisters of Charity', p. 733, p. 734. See [George Robert Gleig], 'The Country Curate. Introduction', *BEM*, 18 (November 1825), 529–40.

128. [Robert Gooch], 'Contagion and Quarantine', *QR*, 27 (July 1822), 524–53 (p. 526); [Robert Gooch], 'Plague, a Contagious Disease', *QR*, 33 (December 1825), 218–57 (p. 218).

129. Robert Gooch to William Blackwood, 2 January 1826, NLS MS 4017, fols 101–2; [Robert Gooch], 'The Quarterly Review of Dr Marmichael on Contagion and the Plague', *BEM*, 19 (February 1826), 130–1.

130. [Robert Ferguson], 'Letters from the Continent. No. I', *BEM*, 16 (November 1824), 555–9 (p. 556).

131. 'Address', *LMG*, 1 (8 December 1827), 1–3 (p. 3).

132. Robert Ferguson to William Blackwood, 15 October 1824, NLS MS 4012, fols 119–20.

133. Robert Ferguson to William Blackwood, [1825?], NLS MS 4014, fols 216–17.

134. Robert Gooch to William Blackwood, 2 January 1826, NLS MS 4017, fols 101–2.

Medical Humanism and *Blackwood's Magazine* at the *Fin de Siècle*

If *Blackwood's* helped to generate a recuperative medical human-ism in the first half of the nineteenth century, what was its legacy? This 'Coda' turns to the *fin de siècle* to trace some key examples of a resurgence of the magazine's mode of medical humanism at a time of perceived crisis for the medical profession, when many began 'to worry that the transformation of medicine into a science, as well as the epistemological and technical successes of the new sciences, may have been bought at too great a price'.[1]

From the mid-nineteenth century, a series of major medico-scientific breakthroughs – most notably in anaesthetics, antisep-tics, and germ theory (with all but the last coming from Scotland) – came to symbolise modern medical progress and the rise of a more 'scientific' medicine.[2] The well-known shift traced by N. D. Jewson, from the bedside medicine of the eighteenth century to the hospital medicine of the post-revolutionary period, had moved forward to the era of laboratory-based medicine, wherein new sciences such as experimental physiology and bacteriology began increasingly to inform clinical medicine.[3] According to Jewson, this 'represented a shift from a person orientated toward an object orientated cosmology', as laboratory-based medicine enabled the medical practitioner 'to conceptualize the sick-man as a material thing to be analysed, and disease as a physico-chemical process to be explained according to the blind inexorable laws of natural science'.[4] In tandem with this, by the end of the century, even *The Lancet* began to express fears that 'a too exclusive professional-ism was growing up among us' and that the '"Doctor" of to-day was not quite so broadly cultured as physicians of the older school were wont to be'.[5]

For Tabitha Sparks, Arthur Conan Doyle's collection of tales *Round the Red Lamp: Being Facts and Fancies of Medical Life* (1894) encapsulates the 'scientization of the doctor' and the medical profession's perceived detachment from what Moir once termed the 'feeling of common humanity'.[6] According to Sparks, this detachment is represented by 'the formal demise of the marriage plot' – fictional doctors no longer experience the traditional narrative resolution of marital bliss by the end of the nineteenth century.[7] She focuses on the tale 'A Physiologist's Wife' and the character Ainslie Grey, chair of physiology at the medical school of Birchespool and 'the very type and embodiment of all that was best in modern science'.[8] Despite disavowing romance as 'the offspring of imagination and of ignorance', Grey determines to recognise 'the great evolutionary instinct which makes either sex the complement of the other' and to marry a beautiful widow, Mrs O'James, only to discover that she is already married to his 'most distinguished pupil'.[9] After encouraging her to reunite with her estranged husband, and declaring his emotional detachment, he nevertheless appears to die of 'what the vulgar would call a broken heart'.[10]

Lawrence Rothfield's study of the development of medical realism through the nineteenth century also culminates with Conan Doyle, but focuses on the famous duo of Sherlock Holmes and Dr John Watson. Rothfield argues that the dominance of Holmes's detective logic – focused on the 'individuated body' rather than the 'embodied person' – represents both the rise of laboratory-based medicine and the new hierarchy between the specialist consultant and the general practitioner (as represented by Watson) that replaced the traditional tripartite medical hierarchy of pre-1858 medicine.[11] As Douglas Kerr astutely indicates, Professor Grey also represents the 'cold consultant':

Written in the age of the triumph of the professions, and of the consulting specialists at their apex (particularly in the clinical domain), [Conan Doyle's] work is everywhere inscribed with both excitement and misgivings about the management of knowledge, a structure of feeling which amounts to nothing less than excitement and misgivings about the direction of modernity itself.[12]

Owen Dudley Edwards sees more misgivings than excitement, viewing Holmes's interpersonal inaptitude as 'throwing into relief the inhumane attitudes towards patients [Conan Doyle] observed at Edinburgh'; he identifies 'human sympathy' as 'the permanent theme of his medical stories in *Round the Red Lamp*'.[13] Aptly then, a modern edition of the collection, edited by Alvin E. Rodin and Jack D. Key, prefaces the title as 'Conan Doyle's Tales of Medical Humanism and Values'.

Intriguingly for my own study, 'A Physiologist's Wife', the first tale of *Round the Red Lamp* to appear in print, was published in *Blackwood's* in September 1890. Conan Doyle was a longtime admirer of *Blackwood's* and had a 'virtual obsession' with appearing within its pages.[14] He submitted the tale 'The Haunted Grange of Goresthorpe – a True Ghost Story' as early as 1877, only to be rejected, a pattern that repeated itself over the next decade for 'The Actor's Duel', 'The Great Keinplatz Experiment', 'Uncle Jeremy's Household', and 'The Surgeon of Gaster Fell'.[15] Despite the magazine's decline in profits at the end of the century,[16] its cultural clout was clearly sustained, and Conan Doyle enthusiastically wrote to William Blackwood III (editor from 1879) that 'as an Edinburgh man my ambition has always been to contribute to the pages of maga'.[17]

There is a pleasing sense of cultural continuity in Conan Doyle's collection of medico-popular tales originating in *Blackwood's*.[18] In the tale 'A Medical Document', he pays tribute to his Blackwoodian predecessor, Samuel Warren, declaring that the 'ablest chronicler of [medical men's] experiences in our literature was a lawyer',[19] while a critic writing for *The Speaker* notes that 'Mr. Doyle is the first writer of fiction of any eminence since the days of Samuel Warren who has made serious use of the experiences of a medical man as a basis for fictitious tales.'[20] (Clearly the texts I identify in the section on 'The Real Physicians' Diaries' were not to the critic's taste.) However, Conan Doyle's character Professor Grey – who at one point responds to his lover's tearful outburst by declaring, 'Your nerves are shaken. Some little congestion of the medulla and pons. It is always constructive to reduce psychic or emotional conditions to their physical equivalents' – has little in common with Warren's neo-Mackenzian late physician.[21] Rather, like Dr Horace Selby of 'The Third Generation' and the surgeon Douglas Stone in 'The Case of Lady Sannox', he serves as a counterpoint to the more humanistic medical men in Conan Doyle's collection, such as Dr Winter in 'Behind the Times'.

In the context of *Blackwood's* in September 1890, the tale builds on a critique of Darwinian materialism that echoes the magazine's earlier critique of political economy as the unfeeling science. At the turn of the century it is now Darwinism and vivisection that come under attack for advancing progress at the price of common humanity – a common humanity which for *Blackwood's* included a continued attunement to religious feelings and aesthetic pleasure. Citing Darwin's own description of his mental transformation, a reviewer of *The Life and Letters of Charles Darwin* (1887) for *Blackwood's* affirms that 'to lose the perception of the beautiful both in art and nature; and to hope for nothing better than to become "a machine for grinding general laws out of large collections of fact," is an appalling progress'.[22] However, while *Blackwood's* lambasts Darwin for having 'spoilt his intelligence with slimy researches into hidden things' and thus, by his own admission, being 'no longer capable of art, poetry, or music', Conan Doyle's tale questions this simple dichotomy.[23] Professor Grey claims indifference to the sublime sensations of the natural world, but when a Mrs Esdaile accuses him of having 'no eye for beauty', Mrs O'James responds, '"On the contrary," ... with a saucy little jerk of her head, "He has just asked me to be his wife."'[24] Ultimately, Grey's death of a broken heart in the denouement of the tale illustrates 'how hard it is to rise above one's humanity'.[25] As with the case of the earlier medical authors in *Blackwood's*, Conan Doyle's contribution works towards healing the perceived 'opposition between literature, aesthetics, and feeling, on the one hand; and science, utility, and reason, on the other'.[26] Even the coldest of consultants is at some level connected to the 'feeling of common humanity'.[27]

At the *fin de siècle Blackwood's* still represented a value system in tension with a scientifically reductive medicine. However, medical contributors such as Conan Doyle remained eager to contribute. To provide just one more brief example: Sir Thomas Grainger Stewart (1837–1900), physician-in-ordinary to Queen Victoria in Scotland from 1882 and president of the Royal College of Physicians of Edinburgh from 1889 to 1891, published his Harveian Oration, 'Notes on Scottish Medicine in the Days of Queen Mary', in *Blackwood's* in June 1893.[28] The annual Harveian Orations were typically published in the *Edinburgh Medical Journal*, but writing to Blackwood, Stewart expresses his preference for it to appear in Maga 'rather than in a medical journal directed to purely professional matters'.[29] On receiving favourable feedback, Stewart waxes lyrical:

> your magazine has always been a prime favourite with me since early boyhood when I used to devour Tom Cringle's Log and 'the old maid and the gun' and such like articles, among the old numbers that had accumulated in my father's house.[30]

In contrast to earlier medical contributors, Stewart had no qualms about his name appearing with his article, nor with a subsequent article, 'Our Duty in Regard to Vaccination'. Likewise, Conan Doyle went so far as to 'stipulate that my name should be attached to ['A Physiologist's Wife'] when it does appear'.[31] This is in tune with a shift away from anonymity in periodical publishing, a rise in the perceived respectability of the author, and also, importantly, a higher valuation of the medical author and his participation in wider culture at the *fin de siècle*.

A survey of the *Edinburgh Medical Journal* (formed via the union of the *Edinburgh Medical and Surgical Journal* and the *Monthly Journal of Medicine*) between 1885 and 1900 reveals the editors' eagerness to review the work of Scottish physician-authors, including not only their personal reminiscences but also novels and poetry, such as a book of verse by Bryan Charles Waller, the Edinburgh medical man responsible for pushing Conan Doyle towards a medical career.[32] The review of his *Perseus with the Hesperides* (1893) characteristically focuses on his place within Edinburgh medical culture:

> Those of us who remember his eager, cultured face, his fine old-world courtesy, his eighteenth century manner, will feel no surprise in recognising our old friend the Lecturer on Pathology and Thesis Gold Medallist in the poet and word-painter.[33]

Literary culture informs this rhetorical performance of collective identity. In April 1890 an obituary for Dr Henry Scott Anderson of Selkirk declares him 'one of the most notable of "Our Gideon Grays,"' while the life and works of Dr John Brown, Edinburgh GP and author of 'Rab and his Friends' (1858), and Oliver Wendell

Holmes (who visited Edinburgh in 1886) are key features.[34] A nostalgia for the Scots language is also pervasive: the publication of a 'Canticle Sung at the Annual Dinner of the Scottish Midland Western Medical Association, Glasgow, 11th October 1889 (1489?)', which parodies Hogg's 'Come all ye jolly shepherds' as 'Cum al ye jollie Doctouris', is an especially striking example.[35] Christopher North even makes an appearance in a review of *The Musings of a Medical* (1891): 'Some of us remember how Christopher North, on one of his gayest holidays, had a kind thought for the dulness [sic] and solitude of the lot of the skeleton hanging in Dr Munro's anatomy class-room.'[36] These nostalgic literary articles and asides, characteristic of the mood at the *fin de siècle*, are intermixed with cutting-edge medico-scientific articles, but overall this is a very different medical journal than that launched by Duncan junior in 1805.

Christopher Lawrence, in a response to S. E. D. Shortt's work on the importance of the 'rhetoric of science' in the professionalisation of medicine, argues that the culture of the gentleman physician continued through at least the end of the nineteenth century – often in conflict with 'scientific' medicine – and was constructed via a rhetoric which emphasised 'that only the gentleman, broadly educated, and soundly educated in the classics, could be equipped for the practice of medicine'.[37] I wish to re-emphasise (without overstating political binaries) that, if the *Edinburgh Review* in its early years provided a natural medium for the type of Whiggish, scientifically-oriented medical culture most often associated with nineteenth-century Scottish medicine, *Blackwood's*, the most influential literary magazine in Scotland in the nineteenth century, provided a natural place for medical men with literary ambitions and Tory sentiments to turn. Some represented, or aspired to join, a gentlemanly, elite medical culture (Robert Gooch and Robert Ferguson perhaps being the best examples of this); or at least, as was the case for Moir and Macnish, they aspired to rise above that 'set of dull dogs' who are 'perfectly contemptible on every subject not immediately connected with pills and potions'.[38] However, the magazine was neither 'anti-science' nor 'anti-medical' in any straightforward sense; rather, as I have attempted to show in this study, it variously enforced, explored, and challenged the growing divide between literary and medico-scientific cultures.

If the *Edinburgh Medical Journal* evinced a nostalgic, nationalistic rhetoric that particularly evoked literary culture, in a period of
intensified interest in national identity, Scottish medicine was not
neglected in *Blackwood's*. In fact, it appears to have been particularly suited to the mode of national identity formation exercised
by the 'Kailyard School' at the *fin de siècle*. Margaret Oliphant's
review of J. M. Barrie's *A Window in Thrums* (1889) for *Blackwood's* is considered a key step in the identification of the Kailyard
(a term not coined until 1895, although retrospectively applied to
Wilson's work by early critics)[39] as 'a national school of Scottish
fiction', characterised by a focus on 'rural and domestic themes'
and the centrality of the Kirk in the community.[40] Oliphant's earlier
review of *The Life of Sir Robert Christison* (1885) in *Blackwood's*
already contains some Kailyard formulations. While eschewing the
rural in favour of the city of Edinburgh, Oliphant emphasises Christison's connection to his locality and the 'advantages of continuity':
'[t]he man who is so entirely representative of the place, and the
place which so fitly, with such hereditary appropriateness, enframes
the man, enhance and set off each other'.[41] This statement might
be read as the narrative impetus behind Maclaren's *A Doctor of
the Old School* (1895), which was extracted from *Beside the Bonnie Brier Bush* (1894), one of the emblematic texts of the Kailyard
School. The episodic novel focuses on Dr William Maclure, the selfless 'Doctor of Drumtochty', who rides day and night and through
all the seasons on his faithful mare, Jess, to care for those living
in the rural Perthshire glen of Drumtochty. 'Weelum', like Christison, has the advantages of a 'hereditary connection', and becomes
a medium for revealing the character of the people of Drumtochty
– defined by a constitutional hardiness, shaped by the rugged land-
scape, and a kindliness and devotion to community, often disguised
by gruffness or cynicism, but revealed by their actions and a certain
look 'in their een'.[42]

Christison, however, 'the natural representative of a culture and
science which have always carried, so to speak, a sprig of heather in
their learned bonnet, and been of Edinburgh first, and after of the
world', is a fit representative of Edinburgh's progressive medico-
scientific culture. According to Oliphant his autobiography reveals
the stark distinction between this culture and Edinburgh's literary culture.[43] While 'Sir Walter himself was about Edinburgh

streets at this time' and 'Christopher North was at the height of his career', there 'was another section of life as vivacious, as full of keen intellectual vitality, pursuing learning upon the same oatmeal, yet scarcely touched by that flood and fullness of literary inspiration which seems to us to fill up all the available space'.[44] This 'section of life' is no less vital a component of Scottish identity, as the *Blackwood's* review of Ella Hill Burton Rodger's *Aberdeen Doctors at Home and Abroad: The Narrative of a Medical School* (1893) insists: '[t]he Scot has a genius for getting on in the world, and has always been specially successful in medicine and surgery'.[45]

Maclaren's sole contribution to *Blackwood's* works towards a reconciliation between what I have termed the 'medical kailyard' and progressive medico-scientific culture. If Warren's *Passages from the Diary of a Late Physician* may be seen as a precursor to Conan Doyle's *Round the Red Lamp*, Moir's suggestion to Blackwood that, in order to extend Wilson's *Lights and Shadows of Scottish Life* (1822), 'The visits of a Country Doctor to his patients might also afford some traits of humourous [sic] peculiarity', appears prophetic of *A Doctor of the Old School*.[46] It is thus another case of pleasing cultural continuity that when Maclaren was invited to submit a 'short study' to *Blackwood's*, he chose to continue the medical portion of *Beside the Bonnie Brier Bush*.[47] The tale, 'A Master of Deceit', which appeared in September 1895 and was subsequently republished as 'How She Came Home' in *The Days of Auld Langsyne* (1895), takes the reader out of the Glen and to London, directly into the home of an elite consulting physician. The narrative turns on Jamie Soutar's attempt to bring the servant lass Lily Grant back to the Glen from London after he hears that she has been ill. When he arrives in London, he is furious to discover that Lily has been sent to a hospital after catching scarlet fever while caring for her employer's children; 'his wrath had no restraint' when he next discovers that she has been taken from the hospital to the home of 'Sir Andrew', the hospital's 'visiting physician'.[48] These actions represent a violation of the values of the 'self-supporting' community, idealised throughout Maclaren's fiction;[49] however, Jamie is appeased when he finds Sir Andrew to be a Scotchman 'with the manner of a great heart', who has taken kindly to Lily for being 'from my country'.[50] Sir Andrew is not unlike Jamie himself, who pretends to be in London 'lookin' aifter some o' Drumsheugh's fat cattle that he sent aff tae the London market' rather than on a journey just for Lily.[51] When Jamie tries to thank him for protecting her from 'the horror of dying in a public place', Sir Andrew responds by disavowing his good deed as 'medical selfishness', asserting that 'I wanted to study Lily's case, and it was handier to have her in my house.'[52] Progressive medico-scientific culture turns out to be a façade for a medical humanism with nationalistic undertones, and the tale shifts the focal point of medical practice from the hospital back to the bedside. Further, Jamie's explicit comparison of Sir Andrew to 'Weelum MacLure' expands the idealisation of the selfless country doctor to the realm of the elite hospital consultant. Jamie responds to Sir Andrew's 'medical selfishness' with characteristic cynicism: 'We hev a doctor in orr pairish that's juist yir marra [equal], aye practeesin' on the sick fouk, an' for lookin' aifter himsel he passes belief.' And he reflects: 'London or Drumtochty, great physeecian or puir country doctor, there's no ane o' them tae mend anither for doonricht gudeness.'[53] In his definitive study of the Kailyard Andrew Nash rightly emphasises that Maclure is 'presented as the very model of a type that no longer exists'; however, I would add that 'A Master of Deceit' encourages an expansion of the 'Godly Commonwealth' to include more modern types of practitioners, and the same goes for the portrayal of the surgical consultant Sir George in *A Doctor of the Old School*.[54]

As Thomas D. Knowles has indicated, the Kailyard was 'designed to promote a moral ethos' and to counter the 'ungodly' literature of Zola, Wilde, and Ibsen in the 1890s.[55] The 'medical kailyard' should be read as likewise driven by a reactionary moral ethos, in presenting a sentimental counterpoint to the cold consultants, heartless vivisectionists, and sinister bodysnatchers of *fin-de-siècle* literature – a counterpoint in demand by the medical profession itself. In his preface to *A Doctor of the Old School* Maclaren testifies to receiving letters 'in commendation of Weelum MacLure' from 'doctors who had received new courage' from reading of the 'Doctor of Drumtochty',[56] and his return to a medical theme in 'A Master of Deceit' may have been in part inspired by this positive reception. In this cultural climate, it is perhaps unsurprising that the centenary of Moir's birth in 1898 brought the medical poet and proto-Kailyard figure newfound popularity with the medical profession.

In December 1897 *The Lancet* announced plans for marking the centenary on the 5th of January: 'the day has been fitly chosen by a number of leading men in Scottish science and literature to commemorate the "beloved physician" and "tender poet" whose life was a beautiful commentary on the "Songs of the Affections" wherein he was a master'.[57] This coverage forms part of a wider celebration of literary medical men in the journal at this time. Moir's sonnet 'The Hospice of St. Bernard' was singled out for praise in 1891, and he is mentioned in an address by 'Dr. Richardson on Medical Poets' in 1885, a general article on 'Medicine and Letters' in 1894, and in a review of John A. Goodchild's *Somnia Medici* in 1893, which shows 'how naturally the medical man may develop into "the singer" – given the true heart that determined him to the most humanitarian of all professions and the fine sense of the beautiful that belongs to every genuine student of the cosmos, moral and material'.[58] In the month prior to the centenary, the medical journal also announced plans to establish a 'Moir Prize', and expressed a desire that Moir's role as a medical historian be considered in the criteria of the literary competition:

> The connexion between literature and the healing art in their concurrent bearing on the evolution of humanity, its 'sorrows and its aspirations,' its achievements and its joys might form no inappropriate theme of the prize in contemplation and might one day inspire some exceptionally gifted competitor to embody in lasting prose or verse the spirit of the 'medical poet' which breathes so warmly from his own sonnet on 'The Hospice of S. Bernard'.[59]

Upon the successful inauguration of the competition, the journal notes that the primary orator of the day, Professor David Masson (1822–1907), has taken the hint in being 'at pains to show the many-sided culture attained by his hero'; it concludes with a reflection on the value of '[s]uch personalities as Dr. Moir's . . . as a stimulating and salutary social leaven'.[60]

The assumptions underlying this celebration of the 'medical poet' will not be unfamiliar to contemporary scholars in the medical humanities. More broadly, the type of medical humanism constructed in *Blackwood's* in the first half of the nineteenth century, and which is again prevalent at the *fin de siècle*, looks forward to the primary roles (to date) of the medical humanities. In a recent special issue of the journal *Medical Humanities* William Viney, Felicity Callard, and Angela Woods polemically argue that the medical humanities have been '(too) often characterised by a dogged focus on the limitations of biomedical knowledge, and how the humanities might bring empathy to clinical practice if allowed adequate epistemological space'. They designate two 'common narratives of purpose': that of the 'utilitarian' companion, intended to support and humanise biomedicine; and, conversely, that of critique, intended 'to disrupt, broaden and embellish what are taken to be the overly reductive, materialist and scientistic definitions of human experience promoted by biomedicine'.[61] My examination of medical contributors to *Blackwood's* has shown how these two roles developed concurrently in one specific, generically experimental and ideologically loaded cultural context. If the Gothic subjectivities of the tale of terror at times anticipate the contemporary critique of biomedical reductionism, the discussion of literary medical men in the 'Noctes' of August 1830 reads as prophetic of the pedagogical ambitions of the medical humanities, while Warren's late physician is a nineteenth-century practitioner of 'Narrative Medicine', and William Pulteney Alison an early advocate for the mode of social medicine still valorised today in Scotland.

If anything, *Blackwood's* mode of medical humanism was further consolidated during the cultural crisis of the *fin de siècle*, while the medical profession expressed congruent sentiments, drawing upon similar rhetorical tropes, in the mainstream professional journals. It is thus unsurprising that in our current crisis contemporary medical humanists have republished both *Round the Red Lamp* and *A Doctor of the Old School* with the avowed mission to emphasise 'the need to counteract the sterility of rampant medical technology with a humanistic orientation to patients' and provide 'valuable tools for any modern physician to rely on'.[62] However, at the same time, proponents of a 'Critical Medical Humanities' are highlighting the 'need to reflect upon the given norms, procedures and values of our medical humanities research community'.[63] Thus, beyond what the present book may have contributed to our understanding of the Romantic ideology of *Blackwood's*, its relationship to medical culture, and the synergistic nature of literature and medicine in the nineteenth-century periodical press,

I hope that it has also shown how politicised and contextually sensitive – how dually problematic and productive – medical humanism has the potential to be.

Notes

1. Huisman and Warner, 'Medical Histories', p. 10; for a summation of this perceived crisis, see MacLeod, 'The "Bankruptcy of Science" Debate'.
2. Corfield, *Power and the Professions in Britain*, p. 140; Lawrence, *Medicine in the Making of Modern Britain*, pp. 55–8; Bynum, 'Medicine in the Laboratory', in *Science and the Practice of Medicine in the Nineteenth Century*, pp. 92–117.
3. For an overview, see Cunningham and Williams (eds), *The Laboratory Revolution in Medicine*.
4. Jewson, 'The Disappearance of the Sick-man from Medical Cosmology', p. 232, p. 238.
5. 'The "Spectator" on "Doctors"', *The Lancet* (31 October 1885), 820.
6. Sparks, *The Doctor in the Victorian Novel*, p. 158; Moir, *The Modern Pythagorean*, vol. 1, p. 123.
7. Ibid. p. 158.
8. A. Conan Doyle, 'A Physiologist's Wife', *BEM*, 148 (September 1890), 339–51 (p. 339).
9. Ibid. p. 344, p. 343, p. 341.
10. Ibid. p. 351.
11. Rothfield, *Vital Signs*, p. 134.
12. Kerr, *Conan Doyle*, p. 56.
13. Edwards, *The Quest for Sherlock Holmes*, p. 200.
14. Ibid. p. 184.
15. Ibid. pp. 183–4.
16. Finkelstein, *The House of Blackwood*, pp. 96–7.
17. Arthur Conan Doyle to William Blackwood, III, undated, NLS MS 4731, fols 55–6.
18. The collection as a whole was subsequently inspired by Jerome K. Jerome's request in 1892 for a series of stories for *The Idler* that might rival the popularity of the Sherlock Holmes series in *The Strand*. See Richard Lancelyn Green and John Michael Gibson, *A Bibliography of A. Conan Doyle* (Oxford: Clarendon Press, 1983), pp. 82–3.
19. Doyle, *Round the Red Lamp*, p. 200.
20. *The Speaker: The Liberal Review*, 10 (December 1894), 605–6 (p. 605).

21. Doyle, 'A Physiologist's Wife', p. 344.
22. 'The Old Saloon', *BEM*, 143 (January 1888), 104–27 (p. 113). For a portrayal of a vivisectionist that echoes the essay on phrenology cited in Chapter 2 (p. 36), see [George Francis Jenner], 'A Philanthropist. A Tale of the Vigilance Committee at San Francisco', *BEM*, 145 (February 1889), 263–79.
23. 'The Old Saloon', *BEM*, 147 (March 1890), 408–28 (p. 417).
24. Doyle, 'A Physiologist's Wife', p. 345.
25. Ibid. p. 349.
26. Connell, *Romanticism, Economics, and the Question of 'Culture'*, p. 11.
27. Moir, *The Modern Pythagorean*, vol. 1, p. 123.
28. George Stronach (rev. Patrick Wallis), 'Stewart, Sir Thomas Grainger (1837–1900)', in *ODNB*, available at http://www.oxforddnb.com/view/article/26509 (last accessed 20 June 2016).
29. Sir T. G. Stewart to William Blackwood, III, 18 May 1893, NLS MS 4607, fols 182–3.
30. Sir T. G. Stewart to William Blackwood, III, 1 June [1893], NLS MS 4607, fols 184–5.
31. Arthur Conan Doyle to William Blackwood, III, 3 April 1890, NLS MS 4550, fols 47–8.
32. Lycett, *Conan Doyle*, p. 43.
33. '[Review of] *Perseus with the Hesperides*. By Bryan Charles Waller. London: George Bell & Son: 1893', *Edinburgh Medical Journal*, 38 (May 1893), 1044–5 (p. 1045).
34. 'Obituary. Henry Scott Anderson, Esq. M.D., F.R.C.S. Edin.', *Edinburgh Medical Journal*, 35 (April 1890), 979–82 (p. 979); 'DR JOHN BROWN: His Life and Work; with Narrative Sketches of JAMES SYME in the Old Minto House Hospital and Dispensary Days; Being the Harveian Society Festival Oration, delivered 11th April 1890. By Alexander Peddie, M.D., F.R.C.P. Ed.', *Edinburgh Medical Journal*, 35 (May, June 1890), 1048–62, 1148–62; 'Obituary. Philip Whiteside Maclagan, M.D.', *Edinburgh Medical Journal*, 38 (July 1892), 100–4 (pp. 100–1); '[Review of] *Recollections of Dr John Brown, author of "Rab and his Friends," etc., with a Selection from his Correspondence*. By Alexander Peddie, M.D., F.R.C.P. Ed., F.R.S.E. London: Perceval & Co.: 1893', *Edinburgh Medical Journal*, 38 (June 1893), 1142; 'Medical News', *Edinburgh Medical Journal*, 32 (August 1886), 188.
35. 'Canticle Sung at the Annual Dinner of the Scottish Midland Western Medical Association, Glasgow, 11th October 1889 (1489?)', *Edinburgh Medical Journal*, 35 (December 1889), 588.

36. '[Review of] *The Musings of a Medical*. No. 1. Edinburgh: James Thin: 1891', *Edinburgh Medical Journal*, 37 (August 1891), 165.

37. Lawrence, 'Incommunicable Knowledge', p. 504, p. 505.

38. Robert Macnish to D. M. Muir, 2 October 1827, NLS Acc. 9856, No. 49.

39. On Wilson's *Lights and Shadows of Scottish Life* as 'pure "Kailyard"', see Millar, *A Literary History of Scotland*, p. 511.

40. Nash, *Kailyard and Scottish Literature*, p. 18, p. 22.

41. [Margaret Oliphant], 'A Scotch Physician', *BEM*, 138 (November 1885), 669–90 (p. 671).

42. Maclaren, *A Doctor of the Old School*, p. 38, p. 189.

43. [Oliphant], 'A Scotch Physician', p. 671.

44. Ibid. p. 676.

45. [Alexander Innes Shand], 'Aberdeen and Aberdeen Doctors', *BEM,* 153 (March 1893), 425–40 (p. 433).

46. D. M. Moir to William Blackwood, 3 March [1822?], NLS MS 4009, fols 106–7.

47. John Watson to William Blackwood, III, 10 April 1895, NLS MS 4640, fols 5–6; see also letters of 20 July 1895, 27 July 1895, 14 August 1895, 4 September 1895, 26 September 1895, NLS MS 4640, fols 7–16.

48. Ian Maclaren, 'A Master of Deceit', *BEM*, 158 (September 1895), 333–40 (p. 335).

49. Nash, *Kailyard and Scottish Literature*, p. 155.

50. Maclaren, 'A Master of Deceit', p. 335, p. 336.

51. Ibid. p. 336.

52. Ibid. p. 338.

53. Ibid. p. 338.

54. Nash, *Kailyard and Scottish Literature*, p. 155, p. 142.

55. Thomas D. Knowles, *Ideology, Art, and Commerce: Aspects of Literary Sociology in the Late Victorian Kailyard* (Goteburg: Acta Universitatis Gothoburgensis, 1983), p. 47, as quoted in Nash, *Kailyard and Scottish Literature*, p. 129.

56. Maclaren, *A Doctor of the Old School*, p. 9.

57. 'A Medical Poet', *The Lancet* (18 December 1897), 1608–9 (p. 1608).

58. 'The Hospice of the Great St. Bernard', *The Lancet* (26 September 1891), 730; 'Dr. Richardson on Medical Poets', *The Lancet* (27 June 1885), 1180; Simon Snell, 'Medicine and Letters', *The Lancet* (15 December 1894), 1440–2; '[Review of] *Somnia Medici*. By John A. Goodchild', *The Lancet* (18 March 1893), 594–5 (p. 594).

59. 'A Medical Poet', p. 1609.

60. 'The Centenary of a Medical Poet', *The Lancet* (15 January 1898), 175.

61. Viney, Callard, and Woods, 'Critical Medical Humanities: Embracing Entanglement, Taking Risks', p. 2, p. 3.
62. 'Introduction', in Rodin and Key (eds), *Conan Doyle's Tales of Medical Humanism and Values*, p. 5. This second quote is taken from an advertisement for *Two Scottish Tales of Medical Compassion* (New York: Cosimo Classics, 2011), available at http://www.amazon.com/Two-Scottish-Tales-Medical-Compassion/dp/1616405449 (last accessed 20 June 2016).
63. Viney, Callard, and Woods, 'Critical Medical Humanities: Embracing Entanglement, Taking Risks', p. 3.

Select Bibliography

Please note that this bibliography does not include material from nineteenth-century periodicals, manuscript sources, or electronic materials. Full references are given in the notes for these materials.

Abercrombie, John, *Inquiries Concerning the Intellectual Powers and the Investigation of Truth* (Edinburgh: Waugh and Innes; M. Ogle, Glasgow; W. Curry, Jun. & co., Dublin; and Whittaker, Treacher & Arnot, London, 1830).

Abercrombie, John, *Inquiries Concerning the Intellectual Powers and the Investigation of Truth*, 11th edn (London: John Murray, 1841).

Adams, Alexander Maxwell, *Sketches from Life. By a Physician* (Glasgow: W. R. M'Phun; London: Simpkin, Marshall, & Co., 1835).

Adams, Alexander Maxwell, 'Remarkable Career. A. M. Adams Primus' Ancestry. From the Autobiography left by Dr. A. M. Adams, Primus' (reprinted from *The Hamilton Advertiser and County of Lanark News*).

Adams, Alexander Maxwell, *A Dynasty of Doctors. The Medical History of the Adams Family. By Dr. Alexander Maxwell Adams, of Tibshelf, Derbyshire* (Tibshelf: Adams, 1922).

Adams, Joseph, *An Illustration of Mr. Hunter's Doctrine, Particularly Concerning the Life of the Blood, in Answer to the Edinburgh Review of Mr. Abernethy's Lectures* (London: Printed by W. Thorne, Red Lion Court, Fleet Street, and sold by J. Johnson, St Paul's Church Yard; and J. Callow, Crown Court, Princes Street, Soho, 1814).

Alison, William Pulteney, *Observations on the Management of the Poor in Scotland, and its Effects on the Health of Great Towns*, 2nd edn (Edinburgh: William Blackwood & Sons; London: Thomas Cadell, 1840).

'Biographical Sketch of Robert Macnish, Esq., LL.D.', in Robert Macnish, *The Anatomy of Drunkenness. With a Sketch of the Author's Life*, new edn (Glasgow: M'Phun, 1859), pp. 9–28.

Brodie, Benjamin, *The Works of Sir Benjamin Collins Brodie, With an Auto-biography*, collected and arranged by Charles Hawkins, 3 vols (London: Longman, Green, Longman, Roberts & Green, 1865).

Brown, John, *Horœ Subsecivœ. Locke and Sydenham with Other Occasional Papers* (Edinburgh: Thomas Constable and Co.; London: Hamilton, Adams and Co., 1858).

Clarke, J. F., *Autobiographical Recollections of the Medical Profession* (London: J. & A. Churchill, 1874).

Cockburn, Henry, *Life of Lord Jeffrey with a Selection from his Correspondence*, 2nd edn, 2 vols (Edinburgh: Adam and Charles Black, 1852).

Cockburn, Henry, *Memorials of his Time* (Edinburgh: Adam and Charles Black, 1856).

Coleridge, Samuel Taylor, *On the Constitution of Church and State According to the Idea of Each* (London: J. M. Dent & Son Ltd., 1972 [1830]).

Coleridge, Samuel Taylor, *Biographia Literaria or Biographical Sketches of My Literary Life and Opinions*, in James Engell and W. Jackson Bate (eds), *The Collected Works of Samuel Taylor Coleridge*, Bollingen Series: 75, 2 vols (Princeton: Princeton University Press, 1983; repr. 1984).

Cuthbert, Charles (ed.), *The Life and Correspondence of Robert Southey*, 6 vols (London: Longman, Brown, Green, and Longmans, 1850).

[Dallas, Alexander], *Protestant Sisters of Charity; A Letter Addressed to the Lord Bishop of London, developing a plan for improving the arrangements at present existing for administering medical advice, and visiting the sick poor* (London: Charles Knight, 1826).

De Quincey, Thomas, *The Works of Thomas De Quincey*, 7 vols (London: Pickering & Chatto, 2000).

Douglas, Robert, *Adventures of a Medical Student*, 3 vols (London: Henry Colburn, 1848).

Doyle, Arthur Conan, *Round the Red Lamp: being facts and fancies of medical life* (London: Methuen & Co., 1894).

Duncan, Andrew, *An Account of the Life, Writings, and Character, of the late Dr Alexander Monro Secondus, Delivered as the Harveian Oration at Edinburgh for the year 1818* (Edinburgh: Archibald Constable & Co.; London: Longman, Hurst, Rees, Orme, and Brown; Dublin: John Cumming, Hodge & Macarthur, 1818).

Ellis, Daniel, *Memoir of the Life and Writings of John Gordon* (Edinburgh: Printed for Archibald Constable and Co. and Hurst, Robinson, and Co., London, 1823).

Extracts from the Diary of a Living Physician, edited by L.F.C. (London: Saunders & Otley, 1851).

Findlay, William, *Robert Burns and the Medical Profession* (Paisley and London: Alexander Gardner, 1898).

Gordon, John, *Outlines of Lectures on Physiology* (Edinburgh: William Blackwood; London: T. & G. Underwood, 1817).

Halford, Sir Henry, *Essays and Orations, Read and Delivered at the Royal College of Physicians; to which is added An Account of the Opening of the Tomb of King Charles I* (London: John Murray, 1831).

Halford, Sir Henry, *On the Education and Conduct of a Physician* (London: John Murray, 1834).

Halford, Sir Henry, *On the Deaths of Some Eminent Persons of Modern Times* (London: John Murray, 1835).

Howison, John, *Foreign Scenes and Travelling Recreations*, 2 vols (Edinburgh: Oliver & Boyd; London: Geo. B. Whittaker, 1825).

Howison, John, *Tales of the Colonies*, 2 vols (London: Henry Colburn and Richard Bentley, 1830).

Howison, William, *The Contest of the Twelve Nations; or, a View of the Different Bases of Human Character and Talent* (Edinburgh: Oliver & Boyd; London: Longman, Rees, Orme, Brown & Green, 1826).

Hume, David, *A Treatise of Human Nature* (Harmondsworth: Penguin Books, 1969; repr. 1985).

Johnson, Samuel, *The Lives of the Poets*, 2 vols (London: Printed for F. C. & I. Rivington and for other Proprietors, 1820).

Lives of British Physicians (London: John Murray, 1830).

[Lockhart, John Gibson], *Peter's Letters to his Kinsfolk*, 3 vols (Edinburgh: Blackwood; London: T. Cadell and W. Davies; Glasgow: John Smith and Son, 1819).

Maclaren, Ian, *A Doctor of the Old School*, with illustrations by Frederick C. Gordon (London: Holder & Stoughton, 1895).

Macnish, Robert, *The Anatomy of Drunkenness. An Inaugural Essay* (Glasgow: W. R. M'Phun, 1827).

Macnish, Robert, *The Anatomy of Drunkenness*, 2nd edn (Glasgow: W. R. M'Phun, 1828).

Macnish, Robert, *The Philosophy of Sleep* (Glasgow: W. R. M'Phun, 1830).

Macnish, Robert, *An Introduction to Phrenology, in the Form of Question and Answer, with an Appendix, and Copious Illustrative Notes* (Glasgow: Reid; Edinburgh: Oliver and Boyd, London: Whittaker, 1836).

Moir, David Macbeth, *Outlines of the Ancient History of Medicine; being a view of the progress of the healing art among the Egyptians, Greeks, Romans, and Arabians* (Edinburgh: William Blackwood, 1831).

Moir, David Macbeth (ed.), *The Modern Pythagorean; A Series of Tales, Essays, and Sketches, By the Late Robert Macnish, LL.D. With the Author's Life, By his Friend, D. M. Moir*, 2 vols (Edinburgh: William Blackwood and Sons; London: T. Cadell, 1838).

[Moir, David Macbeth], *Domestic Verses. By Δ* (Edinburgh: Printed by Neill and Co., 1843).

Moir, David Macbeth, *The Poetical Works of David Macbeth Moir*, 2 vols (Edinburgh and London: William Blackwood and Sons, 1852).

Monro, Alexander, *Observations on Crural Hernia* (Edinburgh: Printed for T. N. Longman and O. Rees, Longman, and W. Laing, 1803).

Percival, Thomas, *Medical Ethics: or, a Code of Institutes and Precepts, adapted to the Professional Conduct of Physicians and Surgeons* (Manchester: Printed by S. Russell, for J. Johnson, St Paul's Church Yard, and R. Bickerstaff, Strand, London, 1803).

'Prospectus of a Course of Lectures on Forensic Medicine to be delivered in the Clyde Street Hall, at Four o'clock, on Mondays, Wednesdays, and Fridays during the Winter Term of the Court of Session. By William Dunlop, Surgeon. The Lectures to Commence on Wednesday, 19th November, 1823' (Printed by A. Balfour and Co., 1823).

Redding, Cyrus, *Fifty Years' Recollections, Literary and Personal, with Observations on Men and Things*, 3 vols (London: Charles J. Skeet, 1858).

Ring, John, *The Beauties of the Edinburgh Review, alias the Stinkpot of Literature* (London: Printed for H. D. Symonds and John Hatchard, 1807).

[Rymer, James Malcolm], *Manuscripts from the Diary of a Physician*, 2 vols (London: E. Lloyd, 1844–7).

Scott, Sir Walter, *The Letters of Sir Walter Scott*, centenary edn, 12 vols (London: Constable & Co., 1932–7).

Seward, Anna, *Anna Seward's Life of Erasmus Darwin*, edited by Philip K. Wilson, Elizabeth A. Dolan, and Malcolm Dick (Studley, Warwickshire: Brewin Books, 2010).

Sketches of Eminent Medical Men (London: The Religious Tract Society, 1847).

Slade, J., *Alice Glynn: A Tale, From the Diary of a Physician. By J. Slade, M.D., K.S.A., M.C.P.* (London: Whittaker and Co., 1845).

Southey, Robert, *Sir Thomas More: or, Colloquies on the Progress and Prospects of Society*, 2 vols (London: John Murray, 1829).

Staples, John, *The Diary of a London Physician* (London: Ward and Lock, 1863).

Stewart, Dugald, *Elements of the Philosophy of the Human Mind*, 3 vols (Edinburgh: Archibald Constable and Company; London: T. Cadell and W. Davies, 1792–1827).

[Thomson, John], *Hints Respecting the Improvement of the Literary & Scientific Education of Candidates for the Degree of Doctor of Medicine in the University of Edinburgh, Humbly Submitted to the Consideration of Patrons and Professors of that Institution; by a Graduate of King's College, Aberdeen* (Edinburgh: Printed for David Brown, St Andrew Street, 1824).

[Thomson, John], *Observations on the Preparatory Education of Candidates for the Degree of Doctor of Medicine, in the Scottish Universities;*

Humbly Submitted to the Consideration of his Majesty's Commissioners for Visiting the Universities and Colleges of Scotland ([N.P.], P. Neill Printer, 1826).

Trotter, Thomas, *An Essay, Medical, Philosophical, and Chemical on Drunkenness and its Effects on the Human Body* (London and New York: Routledge, 1988 [1804]).

[Warren, Samuel], *Affecting Scenes; Being Passages from the Diary of a Physician*, 2 vols (New York: J. & J. Harper, 1831).

[Warren, Samuel], *Passages from the Diary of a Late Physician. With Notes and Illustrations by the Editor*, 2 vols (Edinburgh: William Blackwood; London: T. Cadell, 1832).

Warren, Samuel, 'Preface', in *Passages from the Diary of a Late Physician*, 3 vols, 5th edn (Edinburgh: William Blackwood & Sons; London: T. Cadell, 1838).

Warren, Samuel, 'Preface to the Present Edition', in *Passages from the Diary of a Late Physician*, People's Edition (Edinburgh and London: William Blackwood and Sons, 1854).

Warter, John Wood (ed.), *Selections from the Letters of Robert Southey*, 4 vols (London: Longman, Brown, Green, Longmans & Roberts, 1856).

Welsh, David, *Account of the Life and Writings of Thomas Brown, M.D.* (Edinburgh: W. & C. Tait; London: Longman, Hurst, Rees, Orme, Brown & Green, 1825).

Secondary

Alexander, J. H., '*Blackwood's*: Magazine as Romantic Form', *The Wordsworth Circle*, 15.2 (Spring 1984), pp. 57–68.

Allard, James Robert, *Romanticism, Medicine, and the Poet's Body* (Aldershot and Burlington, VT: Ashgate, 2007).

Allard, James, 'Medicine', in Joel Faflak and Julia M. Wright (eds), *A Handbook of Romanticism Studies* (West Sussex: Wiley-Blackwell, 2012), pp. 375–90.

Atkinson, Dwight, 'The Evolution of Medical Research Writing from 1735 to 1985: The Case of the Edinburgh Medical Journal', *Applied Linguistics*, 13 (1992), pp. 337–74.

Baker, Robert, Dorothy Porter, and Roy Porter (eds), *The Codification of Medical Morality, Historical and Philosophical Studies of the Formalization of Western Medical Morality in the Eighteenth and Nineteenth Centuries. Volume One: Medical Ethics and Etiquette in the Eighteenth Century* (Dordrecht, Boston, and London: Kluwer Academic Publishers, 1993).

Barfoot, Michael, 'Philosophy and Method in Cullen's Medical Teaching', in A. Doig, J. P. S. Ferguson, I. A. Milne, and R. Passmore (eds), *William Cullen and the Eighteenth Century Medical World* (Edinburgh: Edinburgh University Press, 1993), pp. 110–32.

Bewell, Alan, *Romanticism and Colonial Disease* (Baltimore and London: Johns Hopkins University Press, 1999).

Brody, Howard, *Stories of Sickness*, 2nd edn (Oxford: Oxford University Press, 2003).

Brown, Ian, Thomas Owen Clancy, Susan Manning, and Murray G. Pittock (eds), *The Edinburgh History of Scottish Literature, Volume 2: Enlightenment, Britain and Empire (1707–1918)* (Edinburgh: Edinburgh University Press, 2007).

Brown, Michael, *Performing Medicine: Medical Culture and Identity in Provincial England, c.1760–1850* (Manchester and New York: Manchester University Press, 2011).

Budd, Adam, *John Armstrong's The Art of Preserving Health: Eighteenth-Century Sensibility in Practice* (Surrey and Burlington, VT: Ashgate, 2011).

Budge, Gavin (ed.), *Romantic Empiricism: Poetics and the Philosophy of Common Sense, 1780–1830* (Lewisburg: Bucknell University Press, 2007).

Budge, Gavin, 'Medicine, the "manufacturing system," and Southey's Romantic conservatism', *Wordsworth Circle*, 42.1 (2011), pp. 57–63.

Budge, Gavin, *Romanticism, Medicine and the Natural Supernatural: Transcendent Vision and Bodily Spectres, 1789–1852* (Houndmills: Palgrave Macmillan, 2013).

Bynum, W. F., *Science and the Practice of Medicine in the Nineteenth Century* (Cambridge and New York: Cambridge University Press, 1994).

Bynum, W. F., and Roy Porter (eds), *Medical Fringe & Medical Orthodoxy 1750–1850* (London, Sydney, and Wolfebore, NH: Croom Helm, 1987).

Bynum, W. F., Stephen Lock, and Roy Porter (eds), *Medical Journals and Medical Knowledge, Historical Essays* (London and New York: Routledge, 1992).

Cantor, Geoffrey, 'The Academy of Physics at Edinburgh 1797–1800', *Social Studies of Science*, 5 (1975), pp. 109–34.

Cantor, Geoffrey, Gowan Dawson, Graeme Gooday, Richard Noakes, Sally Shuttleworth, and Jonathan R. Topham (eds), *Science in the Nineteenth-Century Periodical: Reading the Magazine of Nature* (Cambridge and New York: Cambridge University Press, 2004).

Chalmers, John (ed.), *Andrew Duncan Senior: Physician of the Enlightenment* (Edinburgh: National Museums Scotland, 2010).

Charon, Rita, *Narrative Medicine: Honoring the Stories of Illness* (Oxford: Oxford University Press, 2006).

Checkland, Olive, 'Chalmers and William Pulteney Alison: A Conflict of Views on Scottish Social Policy' in A. C. Cheyne (ed.), *The Practical and the Pious: Essays on Thomas Chalmers (1780–1847)* (Edinburgh: The Saint Andrews Press, 1985), pp. 130–40.

Chitnis, Anand C., *The Scottish Enlightenment: A Social History* (London: Croom Helm; Totawa, NJ: Rowman and Littlefield, 1976).

Chitnis, Anand C., *The Scottish Enlightenment & Early Victorian English Society* (London, Sydney, Dover, New Hampshire: Croom Helm, 1986).

Christie, William, *The Edinburgh Review and the Literary Culture of Romantic Britain: Mammoth and Megalonyx* (London: Pickering & Chatto, 2009).

Class, Monika, 'Introduction: Medical Case Histories as Genre: New Approaches', *Literature and Medicine*, 32.1 (Spring 2014), pp. vii–xvi.

Clive, John, *Scotch Reviewers: The Edinburgh Review, 1802–1815* (London: Faber and Faber, 1957).

Comrie, John, *History of Scottish Medicine*, 2nd edn, 2 vols (London: Wellcome History of Medicine Museum, 1932).

Connell, Phillip, *Romanticism, Economics, and the Question of 'Culture'* (Oxford: Oxford University Press, 2001).

Corfield, Penelope J., *Power and the Professions in Britain 1700–1850* (London and New York: Routledge, 1995).

Coyer, Megan, 'The Medical Kailyard', *The Bottle Imp* 15 (2014), available at http://www.arts.gla.ac.uk/ScotLit/ASLS/SWE/TBI/TBIIssue15/Coyer.pdf (last accessed 15 June 2016).

Coyer, Megan J., and David E. Shuttleton (eds), *Scottish Medicine and Literary Culture, 1726–1832* (Amsterdam and New York: Rodopi, 2014).

Craig, David M., *Robert Southey and Romantic Apostasy: Political Argument in Britain, 1780–1840* (Suffolk: Royal Historical Society and the Boydell Press, 2007).

Crawford, Catherine, 'A scientific profession: medical reform and forensic medicine in British periodicals of the early nineteenth century', in Roger French and Andrew Wear (eds), *British Medicine in an Age of Reform* (London and New York: Routledge, 1991), pp. 203–30.

Crowther, M. Anne, and Brenda White, *On Soul and Conscience: the Medical Expert and Crime* (Aberdeen: Aberdeen University Press, 1988).

Cunningham, Andrew, and Perry Williams (eds), *The Laboratory Revolution in Medicine* (Cambridge and New York: Cambridge University Press, 1992).

Cutmore, Jonathan (ed.), *Conservativism and the Quarterly Review: A Critical Analysis* (London: Pickering & Chatto, 2007).

Cutmore, Jonathan, *Contributors to the Quarterly Review: A History, 1809–25* (London: Pickering & Chatto, 2008).

Daffron, Benjamin Eric, *Romantic Doubles: Sex and Sympathy in British Gothic Literature 1790–1830* (New York: AMS Press, 2002).

Damasio, Antonio, *Looking for Spinoza: Joy, Sorrow, and the Feeling Brain* (Orlando: Harcourt Brace International, 2003).

Daston, Lorraine, and Peter Galison, *Objectivity* (New York: Zone Books, 2007).

Davie, George E., *The Scottish Enlightenment and Other Essays* (Edinburgh: Polygon, 1991).

Desmond, Adrian, *The Politics of Evolution: Morphology, Medicine, and Reform in Radical London* (Chicago and London: The University of Chicago Press, 1989).

Dingwall, Helen M., *A History of Scottish Medicine* (Edinburgh: Edinburgh University Press, 2003).

Duncan, Ian, '*Blackwood's* and Romantic Nationalism', in David Finkelstein (ed.), *Print Culture and the Blackwood Tradition: 1805–1930* (Toronto: University of Toronto Press, 2006), pp. 70–89.

Duncan, Ian, *Scott's Shadow: The Novel in Romantic Edinburgh* (Princeton: Princeton University Press, 2007).

Duncan, Ian, 'Hume and the Scottish Enlightenment', in Ian Brown, Thomas Owen Clancy, Susan Manning, and Murray G. Pittock (eds), *The Edinburgh History of Scottish Literature, Volume 2: Enlightenment, Britain and Empire (1707–1918)* (Edinburgh: Edinburgh University Press, 2007), pp. 71–9.

Eastwood, David, 'Robert Southey and the Intellectual Origins of Romantic Conservatism', *The English Historical Review*, 104.411 (April 1989), pp. 308–31.

Edwards, Owen Dudley, *The Quest for Sherlock Holmes: A Biographical Study of Arthur Conan Doyle* (Edinburgh: Mainstream Publishing, 1983).

Emerson, Roger L., *Essays on David Hume, Medical Men and the Scottish Enlightenment, 'Industry, Knowledge and Humanity'* (Farnham and Burlington, VT: Ashgate, 2009).

Faubert, Michelle, *Rhyming Reason: The Poetry of Romantic-Era Psychologists* (London: Pickering & Chatto, 2009).

Fetter, Frank W., 'The Economic Articles in the *Quarterly Review* and Their Authors, 1809–1852, I', *Journal of Political Economy*, 66.1 (February 1958), pp. 47–64.

Fetter, Frank W., 'The Economic Articles in *Blackwood's Edinburgh Magazine* and their Authors, 1817–1853, Part I', *Scottish Journal of Political Economy*, 7.1 (February 1960), pp. 85–107.

Fetter, Frank W., 'Economy Controversy in the British Reviews, 1802–1850', *Economica*, New Series, 32.128 (November 1965), pp. 424–37.

Finkelstein, David, *The House of Blackwood: Author-Publisher Relations in the Victorian Era* (University Park: University of Pennsylvania Press, 2002).

Fisher, Judith L., '"In the Present Famine of Anything Substantial": *Fraser's* "Portraits" and the Construction of Literary Celebrity; Or, "Personality, Personality Is the Appetite of the Age"', *Victorian Periodicals Review*, 39.2 (Summer 2006), pp. 97–135.

Flynn, Philip, *Enlightenment Scotland* (Edinburgh: Scottish Academic Press, 1992).

Fontana, Biancamaria, *Rethinking the Politics of Commercial Society: The Edinburgh Review, 1802–1832* (Cambridge and New York: Cambridge University Press, 1985).

Foucault, Michel, *The Birth of the Clinic: An Archaeology of Medical Perception*, trans. A. M. Sheridan (London and New York: Routledge, 1989).

Furst, Lillian, 'Struggling for Medical Reform in Middlemarch', *Nineteenth-Century Literature*, 48.3 (December 1993), pp. 341–61.

Graham, W. H., *The Tiger of Canada West* (Toronto and Vancouver: Clarke, Irwin & Company, 1962).

Gray, Robert, *The Factory Question and Industrial England, 1830–1860* (Cambridge and New York: Cambridge University Press, 1996).

Grave, S. A., *The Scottish Philosophy of Commonsense* (Oxford: Clarendon Press, 1960).

Green, Richard Lancelyn, and John Michael Gibson, *A Bibliography of A. Conan Doyle* (Oxford: Clarendon Press, 1983).

Guerrini, Anita, 'Alexander Monro *Primus* and the Moral Theatre of Anatomy', *Eighteenth Century*, 47 (2006), pp. 1–18.

Haakonssen, Lisbeth, *Medicine and Morals in the Enlightenment: John Gregory, Thomas Percival, and Benjamin Rush* (Amsterdam and Atlanta: Rodopi, 1997).

Hamilton, David, *The Healers: A History of Medicine in Scotland* (Edinburgh: Canongate, 1981).

Hamilton, David, 'The Scottish Enlightenment and Clinical Medicine', in Derek Dow (ed.), *The Influence of Scottish Medicine: An Historical Assessment of its International Impact* (Carnforth and Park Ridge, NJ: Parthenon Publishing Group, 1988), pp. 103–12.

Hamlin, Christopher, *Public Health and Social Justice in the Age of Chadwick Britain, 1800–1854* (Cambridge and New York: Cambridge University Press, 1998).

Hamlin, Christopher, 'William Pulteney Alison, the Scottish Philosophy, and the Making of a Political Medicine', *Journal of the History of Medicine and Allied Sciences*, 61.2 (April 2006), pp. 144–86.

Hampshire, Stuart, *Spinoza and Spinozism* (Oxford: Clarendon Press, 2005).

Hart, Francis R., *Lockhart as Romantic Biographer* (Edinburgh: Edinburgh University Press, 1971).

Hawkins, Anne Hunsaker, *Reconstructing Illness: Studies in Pathography* (West Lafayette: Purdue University Press, 1993).

Hewitt, Regina, 'Introduction: Observations and Conjectures on John Galt's Place in Scottish Enlightenment and Romantic-era Studies', in Regina Hewitt (ed.), *John Galt: Observations & Conjectures on Literature, History, and Society* (Lewisburg: Bucknell University Press, 2012), pp. 1–32.

Higgins, David, *Romantic Genius and the Literary Magazine: Biography, Celebrity and Politics* (London and New York: Routledge, 2005).

Higgins, David, 'Imaging the Exotic: De Quincey and Lamb in the *London Magazine*', *Romanticism*, 17.3 (2011), pp. 288–98.

Hochel, Matej, and Emilio G. Milán, 'Synaesthesia: The Existing State of Affairs', *Cognitive Neuropsychology*, 25.1 (2008), pp. 93–117.

Holloway, S. W. F., 'Medical Education in England, 1830–1858: A Sociological Analysis', *History* 49 (1964), pp. 299–324.

Huisman, Frank, and John Harley Warner, 'Medical Histories', in Frank Huisman and John Harley Warner (eds), *Locating Medical History: The Stories and Their Meanings* (Baltimore and London: Johns Hopkins University Press, 2006), pp. 1–30.

Jackson, Noel, *Science and Sensation in Romantic Poetry* (Cambridge and New York: Cambridge University Press, 2008).

Jacyna, L. S., *Philosophic Whigs: Medicine, Science, and Citizenship in Edinburgh, 1789–1848* (London and New York: Routledge, 1994).

Jenkinson, Jacqueline, *Scottish Medical Societies, 1731–1939* (Edinburgh: Edinburgh University Press, 1993).

Jewson, N. D., 'Medical Knowledge and the Patronage System in 18th Century England', *Sociology*, 8 (1974), pp. 369–85.

Jewson, N. D., 'The Disappearance of the Sick-man from Medical Cosmology, 1770–1870', *Sociology*, 10.2 (May 1976), pp. 225–44.

Keel, Othmar, 'The Politics of Health and the Institutionalisation of Clinical Practices in Europe in the Second Half of the Eighteenth Century', in W. F. Bynum and Roy Porter (eds), *William Hunter and the Eighteenth-Century Medical World* (Cambridge and New York: Cambridge University Press, 1985), pp. 207–56.

Kennedy, Meegan, *Revising the Clinic: Vision and Representation in Victorian Medical Narrative and the Novel* (Columbus: Ohio State University Press, 2010).

Kennedy, Meegan, 'The Ghost in the Clinic: Gothic Medicine and Curious Fiction in Samuel Warren's "Diary of a Late Physician"', *Victorian Literature and Culture*, 32.3 (2004), pp. 327–51.

Kerr, Douglas, *Conan Doyle: Writing, Profession, and Practice* (Oxford: Oxford University Press, 2013).

Killick, Tim, *British Short Fiction in the Early Nineteenth Century: The Rise of the Tale* (Aldershot and Burlington, VT: Ashgate, 2008).

Klancher, Jon, *The Making of English Reading Audiences, 1790–1832* (Madison: University of Wisconsin Press, 1987).

Larson, Magali Sarfatti, *The Rise of Professionalism: A Sociological Analysis* (Berkeley, Los Angeles, and London: University of California Press, 1977).

Lawrence, Christopher, 'The Nervous System and Society in the Scottish Enlightenment', in B. Barnes and S. Shapin (eds), *Natural Order: Historical Studies of Scientific Culture* (London and Beverly Hills: Sage Publications, 1979), pp. 19–40.

Lawrence, Christopher, 'Incommunicable Knowledge: Science, Technology and the Clinical Art in Britain 1850–1914', *Journal of Contemporary History*, 20.4 (October 1985), pp. 503–20.

Lawrence, Christopher, 'The Edinburgh Medical School and the End of the "Old Thing" 1790–1830', *History of Universities*, 7 (1988), pp. 259–86.

Lawrence, Christopher, *Medicine in the Making of Modern Britain, 1700–1920* (London and New York: Routledge, 1994).

Leary, Patrick, '*Fraser's Magazine* and the Literary Life, 1830–1847', *Victorian Periodicals Review*, 27.2 (Summer 1994), pp. 105–26.

Leask, Nigel, *British Romantic Writers and the East: Anxieties of Empire* (Cambridge and New York: Cambridge University Press, 1992).

Leask, Nigel, *Curiosity and the Aesthetics of Travel Writing, 1770–1840, 'From an Antique Land'* (Oxford: Oxford University Press, 2002).

Leavis, F. R., and Q. D. Leavis, *Dickens the Novelist* (London: Chatto & Windus, 1970).

Ledger, Sally, 'Radical Writing', in Joanne Shattock (ed.), *The Cambridge Companion to English Literature, 1830–1914* (Cambridge and New York: Cambridge University Press, 2010), pp. 127–46.

Lehrer, Keith, 'Beyond Impressions and Ideas: Hume v. Reid', in Peter Jones (ed.), *The 'Science of Man' in the Scottish Enlightenment: Hume, Reid, and their Contemporaries* (Edinburgh: Edinburgh University Press, 1989), pp. 108–23.

Levin, Susan M., *The Romantic Art of Confession: De Quincey, Musset, Sand, Lamb, Hogg, Frémy, Soulié, Janin* (Columbia, SC: Camden House, 1998).

Logan, Peter Melville, *Nerves and Narratives: A Cultural History of Hysteria in 19th-Century British Prose* (Berkeley: University of California Press, 1997).

Loudon, Irvine, *Medical Care and the General Practitioner 1750–1850* (Oxford: Clarendon Press, 1986).

Marshall, Tim, *Murdering to Dissect: Grave-robbing, Frankenstein and the Anatomy Literature* (Manchester and New York: Manchester University Press, 1995).

Martin, Sheenagh M. K., *William Pulteney Alison: activist philanthropist and pioneer of social medicine* (unpublished PhD Thesis, University of St Andrews, 1997).

Mason, Nicolas, '"The Quack Has Become God": Puffery, Print and the "Death" of Literature in Romantic-Era Britain', *Nineteenth-Century Literature*, 60.1 (June 2005), pp. 1–31.

McCracken-Flesher, Caroline, *The Doctor Dissected: A Cultural Autopsy of the Burke and Hare Murders* (Oxford and New York: Oxford University Press, 2012).

McCrae, M., 'Andrew Duncan and the Health of Nations', *Journal of the Royal College of Physicians Edinburgh*, 33 (2003), pp. 2–11.

McCullough, Laurence B., *John Gregory and the Invention of Professional Medical Ethics and the Profession of Medicine* (Dordrecht, Boston, London: Kluwer Academic Publishers, 1998).

McCullough, Laurence B., *John Gregory's Writings on Medical Ethics and Philosophy of Medicine* (Dordrecht, Boston, and London: Kluwer Academic Publishers, 1998).

MacLeod, Roy, 'The "Bankruptcy of Science" Debate: The Creed of Science and its Critics, 1885–1900', *Science, Technology, & Human Values*, 7.41 (Autumn 1982), pp. 2–15.

McMullen, Bonnie Shannon, '"A Wrong Port": Colonial Havana under Northern Eyes', *Journeys*, 7.1 (Summer 2006), pp. 67–80.

Michie, Michael, *An Enlightenment Tory in Victorian Scotland: The Career of Sir Archibald Alison* (East Linton: Tuckwell Press; McGill-Queen's University Press, 1997).

Millar, J. H., *A Literary History of Scotland* (London: T. Fisher Unwin, 1903).

Miller, Stephen, *Three Deaths and Enlightenment Thought: Hume, Johnson, Marat* (Lewisburg: Bucknell University Press; London: Associated University Presses, 2001).

Milligan, Barry, 'Morphine-Addicted Doctors, the English Opium-Eater, and Embattled Medical Authority', *Victorian Literature and Culture*, 33.2 (2005), pp. 541–55.

Milne, J. M., *The Politics of Blackwood's, 1817–1846: A Study of the political, economic, and social articles in Blackwood's Edinburgh*

Magazine and of selected contributors (unpublished PhD thesis, University of Newcastle upon Tyne, November 1984).

Milne, Maurice, 'Archibald Alison: Conservative Controversialist', *Albion: A Quarterly Journal Concerned with British Studies*, 27.3 (Autumn 1995), pp. 419–43.

Morrison, Robert, 'John Howison of 'Blackwood's Magazine'', *Notes and Queries*, 42.2 (June 1995), p. 191.

Morrison, Robert, 'Opium-Eaters and Magazine Wars: De Quincey and Coleridge in 1821', *Victorian Periodicals Review*, 30.1 (Spring 1997), pp. 27–40.

Morrison, Robert, and Chris Baldick, 'Introduction', in Robert Morrison and Chris Baldick (eds), *Tales of Terror from Blackwood's Magazine* (Oxford and New York: Oxford University Press, 1995), pp. vii–xviii.

Morrison, Robert, and Daniel S. Roberts (eds), *Romanticism and Blackwood's Magazine, 'An Unprecedented Phenomenon'* (Houndmills and New York: Palgrave Macmillan, 2013).

Munk, William, *The Roll of the Royal College of Physicians of London; Comprising Biographical Sketches of all the Eminent Physicians, whose names are recorded in the annals, from the foundation of the college in 1518 to its removal in 1825, from Warwick Lane to Pall Mall East. 2nd edition, revised and enlarged, Vol. III., 1801 to 1825* (London: Published by the College, Pall Mall East, 1878).

Nash, Andrew, *Kailyard and Scottish Literature* (Amsterdam and New York: Rodopi, 2007).

Newman, Rebecca Edwards, '"Prosecuting the Onus Criminus": Early Criticism of the Novel in *Fraser's Magazine*', *Victorian Periodicals Review*, 35.4 (Winter 2002), pp. 401–19.

Noble, Andrew, 'John Wilson (Christopher North) and the Tory Hegemony', in Douglas Gifford (ed.), *The History of Scottish Literature, Volume 3, Nineteenth Century* (Aberdeen: Aberdeen University Press, 1988), pp. 125–52.

O'Brien, D. P., *J. R. McCulloch: A Study in Classical Economics* (London: George Allen & Unwin Ltd, 1970).

Parker, Mark, *Literary Magazines and British Romanticism* (Cambridge: Cambridge University Press, 2000).

Parry, Noel, and Jose Parry, *The Rise of the Medical Profession: A Study of Collective Social Mobility* (London: Croom Helm, 1976).

Passmore, Reginald, *Fellows of Edinburgh's College of Physicians during the Scottish Enlightenment* (Edinburgh: Royal College of Physicians of Edinburgh, 2001).

Peterson, M. Jeanne, *The Medical Profession in Mid-Victorian London* (Berkeley: University of California Press, 1978).

Phillipson, Nicholas, 'Towards a Definition of the Scottish Enlightenment', in Paul Fritz and David Williams (eds), *City and Society in the Eighteenth Century* (Toronto: Hakkert, 1973), pp. 125–47.

Phillipson, Nicholas, 'Culture and Society in the Eighteenth-Century Province: The Case of Edinburgh and the Scottish Enlightenment', in Lawrence Stone (ed.), *The University in Society: Studies in the History of Higher Education*, 2 vols (Princeton: Princeton University Press; London: Oxford University Press, 1974), vol. 2, pp. 407–48.

Phillipson, Nicholas, 'The Scottish Enlightenment', in Roy Porter and Mikuláš Teich (eds), *The Enlightenment in National Context* (Cambridge: Cambridge University Press, 1981), pp. 19–40.

Pitman, Joy, 'David M. Moir: Cholera Papers', *Proceedings of the Royal College of Physicians of Edinburgh*, 22 (1992), pp. 543–7.

Pomata, Gianna, 'The Medical Case Narrative: Distant Reading of an Epistemic Genre', *Literature and Medicine*, 32.1 (Spring 2014), pp. 1–23.

Porter, Dorothy, and Roy Porter, *Patient's Progress: Doctors and Doctoring in Eighteenth-Century England* (Cambridge: Polity Press; Oxford: Basil Blackwell, 1989).

Porter, Roy, 'Lay Medical Knowledge in the Eighteenth Century: The Evidence of the *Gentleman's Magazine*', *Medical History*, 29 (1985), pp. 138–68.

Porter, Roy, *Quacks: Fakers & Charlatans in English Medicine* (Stroud: Tempus, 2000 [1989]).

Porter, Roy, *Bodies Politic: Disease, Death and Doctors in Britain, 1650–1900* (London: Reaktion Books, 2001).

Pottinger, George, *Heirs of the Enlightenment: Edinburgh reviewers and writers 1800–1830* (Edinburgh: Scottish Academic Press, 1992).

Richardson, Alan, *British Romanticism and the Science of the Mind* (Cambridge and New York: Cambridge University Press, 2001).

Richardson, Ruth, *Death, Dissection and the Destitute* (London and New York: Routledge & Kegan Paul, 1987).

Risse, Guenter B., 'Historicism in Medical History: Heinrich Damerow's "Philosophical" Historiography in Romantic Germany', *Bulletin of the History of Medicine*, 43 (1969), pp. 201–11.

Risse, Guenter B., 'Kant, Schelling, and the Early Search for a Philosophical "Science" of Medicine in Germany', *Journal of the History of Medicine*, 27 (April 1972), pp. 145–58.

Risse, Guenter B., '"Philosophical" Medicine in Nineteenth-Century Germany: An Episode in the Relations between Philosophy and Medicine', *Journal of Medicine and Philosophy*, 1 (1976), pp. 72–92.

Roberts, David, 'The Social Conscience of Tory Periodicals', *Victorian Periodicals Newsletter*, 10.3 (September 1977), pp. 154–69.

Roberts, Marie Mulvey, and Roy Porter (eds), *Literature & Medicine during the Eighteenth Century* (London and New York: Routledge, 1993).

Rodin, Alvin E., and Jack D. Key (eds), *Conan Doyle's Tales of Medical Humanism and Values: Round the Red Lamp: being facts and fancies of medical life, with other medical short stories* (Malabar, FL: Krieger, 1992).

Roe, Nicolas, *John Keats and the Culture of Dissent* (Oxford: Clarendon Press, 1997).

Rosner, Lisa, *Medical Education in the Age of Improvement: Edinburgh Students and Apprentices, 1760–1826* (Edinburgh: Edinburgh University Press, 1991).

Rosner, Lisa, *The Anatomy Murders: Being the True and Spectacular History of Edinburgh's Notorious Burke and Hare and of the Man of Science Who Abetted Them in the Commission of Their Most Heinous Crimes* (Philadelphia: University of Pennsylvania Press, 2010).

Rothfield, Lawrence, *Vital Signs: Medical Realism in Nineteenth-Century Fiction* (Princeton: Princeton University Press, 1992).

Rothfield, Lawrence, 'Medicine', in Herbert F. Tucker (ed.), *A Companion to Victorian Literature & Culture* (Oxford and Malden, MA: Blackwell Publishers, 1999), pp. 170–82.

Rousseau, G. S., '"Stung into action. . .": Medicine, Professionalism, and the News', *Prose Studies: History, Theory, Criticism*, 21.2 (1998), pp. 176–205.

Ruston, Sharon, *Shelley and Vitality* (Houndmills and New York: Palgrave Macmillan, 2005; repr. 2012).

Ruston, Sharon, *Creating Romanticism: Case Studies in the Literature, Science and Medicine of the 1790s* (Houndmills and New York: Palgrave Macmillan, 2013).

Schoenfield, Mark, *British Periodicals and Romantic Identity: The 'Literary Lower Empire'* (New York and Houndmills: Palgrave Macmillan, 2009).

Shortt, S. E. D., 'Physicians, Science, and Status: Issues in the Professionalisation of Anglo-American Medicine in the Nineteenth Century', *Medical History*, 27 (1983), pp. 51–68.

Sparks, Tabitha, *The Doctor in the Victorian Novel: Family Practices* (Farnham and Burlington, VT: Ashgate, 2009).

Stack, David, *Queen Victoria's Skull: George Combe and the Mid-Victorian Mind* (London: Hambledon Continuum, 2008).

Story, Mark, *Robert Southey: A Life* (Oxford and New York: Oxford University Press, 1997).

Sucksmith, Harvey Peter, 'The Secret of Immediacy: Dickens' Debt to the Tale of Terror in *Blackwood's*', *Nineteenth-Century Fiction*, 26.2 (September 1971), pp. 145–57.

Swann, Elsie, *Christopher North <John Wilson>* (Edinburgh, London: Oliver and Boyd, 1934).

Sweet, Nanora, 'The *New Monthly Magazine* and the Liberalism of the 1820s', in Kim Wheatley (ed.), *Romantic Periodicals and Print Culture* (London, Portland: Frank Cass, 2003), pp. 147–62.

Symonds, Barry, *De Quincey to His Publishers: The Letters of Thomas De Quincey, and Other Letters 1819–1832* (unpublished PhD thesis, University of Edinburgh, 1994).

Temkin, Owsei, 'Basic Science, Medicine, and the Romantic Era', *Bulletin of the History of Medicine*, 38 (1963), pp. 97–129.

Thrall, Miriam M. H., *Rebellious Fraser's, Nol Yorke's Magazine in the Days of Maginn, Thackeray, and Carlyle* (New York: Columbia University Press, 1934).

Trevor-Roper, Hugh, 'The Scottish Enlightenment', *Studies on Voltaire and the Eighteenth Century*, 58 (1967), pp. 1635–58.

Tröhler, Ulrich, *"To Improve the Evidence of Medicine": The 18th Century British Origins of a Critical Approach* (Edinburgh: Royal College of Physicians of Edinburgh, 2000).

van Wyhe, John, *Phrenology and the Origins of Victorian Scientific Naturalism* (Aldershot and Burlington, VT: Ashgate, 2004).

Vickers, Neil, *Coleridge and the Doctors, 1795–1806* (Oxford: Clarendon Press, 2004).

Viney, William, Felicity Callard, and Angela Woods, 'Critical Medical Humanities: Embracing Entanglement, Taking Risks', *Medical Humanities*, 41.1 (June 2015), pp. 2–7.

Waddington, Ivan, *The Medical Profession in the Industrial Revolution* (Dublin: Gill and Macmillan, 1984).

Watson, Katherine D., *Forensic Medicine in Western Society: A History* (London and New York: Routledge, 2011).

Webb, Nick, *Wish You Were Here: The Official Biography of Douglas Adams* (London: Headline, 2003).

White, Brenda, 'Training medical policemen: forensic medicine and public health in nineteenth-century Scotland', in Michael Clark and Catherine Crawford (eds), *Legal Medicine in History* (Cambridge and New York: Cambridge University Press, 1994), pp. 145–64.

Williams, Perry, 'Religion, respectability and the origins of the modern nurse', in Roger French and Andrew Wear (eds), *British Medicine in an Age of Reform* (London and New York: Routledge, 1991), pp. 231–55.

Withers, C. W. J., and Paul Wood (eds), *Science and Medicine in the Scottish Enlightenment* (East Linton: Tuckwell Press, 2002).

Wood, Paul, 'Science in the Scottish Enlightenment', in Alexander Broadie (ed.), *The Cambridge Companion to the Scottish Enlightenment* (Cambridge and New York: Cambridge University Press, 2003), pp. 94–116.

Worthington, Heather, *The Rise of the Detective in Early Nineteenth-Century Fiction* (Houndmills and New York: Palgrave Macmillan, 2005).

Index

EU representative:
Easy Access System Europe
Mustamäe tee 50, 10621 Tallinn, Estonia
Gpsr.requests@easproject.com